Exam
Success

By Lewis Morris

Copyright © Network4Learning, Inc. 2018.

www.insiderswords.com/Success

ISBN-13: 978-1717712066

Table of Contents

What is "Insider Language"?

Recent research has confirmed what we have known for decades: The strongest students and leaders in industry have a mastered an Insider Language in their subject and field. This Insider language is made up of the technical terms and vocabulary necessary to communicate effectively in classes or the workplace. For those who master it, learning is easier, faster, and much more enjoyable.

Most students who are surveyed report that the greatest challenge to any course of study is learning the vocabulary. When we examine typical college courses, we discover that there is, on average, 250 Insider Terms a student must learn over the course of a semester. Further, most exams rely heavily on this set of words for assessment purposes. The structure of multiple choice exams lends itself perfectly to the testing of this Insider Language. Students who can differentiate between Insider Language terms can handle challenging exam questions with ease and confidence.

From recent research on learning and vocabulary we have learned:

- Your knowledge of any subject is contained in the content-specific words you know. The more of these terms that you know, the easier it is to understand and recall important information; the easier it will be to communicate your ideas to peers, professors, supervisors, and co-workers. The stronger your content-area vocabulary is, the higher your scores will be on your exams and written assignments.

- Students who develop a strong Insider Language perform better on tests, learn faster, retain more information, and express greater satisfaction in learning.

- Familiarizing yourself with subject-area vocabulary before formal study (pre-learning) is the most effective way to learn this language and reap the most benefit.

- The vocabulary on standardized exams come directly from the stated objectives of the test-makers. This means that the vocabulary found on standardized exams is predictable. Our books focus on this vocabulary.

- Most multiple-choice exams are glorified vocabulary quizzes. Think about the format of a multiple-choice question. The question stem is a definition of a term and the choices (known as distractors) are 4 or 5 similar words. Your task is to differentiate between the meanings of those terms and choose the correct word.

- It takes a person several exposures to a new word to be able to use it with confidence in conversation or in writing. You need to process these words several different ways to make them part of your long-term memory.

The goals of this book are:
- To give you an "Insider Language" for your subject.
- Pre-teach the most important words before you set out on a traditional course of review or study.
- Teach you the most important words in your subject area.
- Teach you strategies for learning subject-area words on your own.
- Boost your confidence in your ability to master this language and support you in your study.
- Reduce the stress of studying and provide you with fun activities that work.

How it works:
The secret to mastering Insider Language is through repetition and exposure. We have eleven steps for you to follow:

1. Read the word and definition in the glossary out loud. "See it, Say it"
2. Identify the part of speech the word belongs to such as noun, verb, adverb, or adjective. This will help you group the word and identify similar words.
3. Place the word in context by using it in a sentence. Write this sentence down and read it aloud.
4. Use "Chunking" to group the words. Make a diagram or word cloud using these groups.
5. Make connections to the words by creating analogies.
6. Create mnemonics that help you recognize patterns and orders of words by substituting the words for more memorable items or actions.
7. Examine the morphology of the word, that is, identify the root, prefix, and suffix that make up the word. Identify similar and related words.
8. Complete word games and puzzles such as crosswords and word searches.
9. Complete matching questions that require you to differentiate between related words.
10. Complete Multiple-choice questions containing the words.
11. Create a visual metaphor or "memory cartoon" to make a mental picture of the word and related processes.

By completing this word study process, you will be exposed to the terminology in various ways that will activate your memory and create a lasting understanding of this language.

The strategies in this book are designed to make you an independent expert at learning insider language. These strategies include:

- Verbalizing the word by reading it and its definition aloud ("See It, Say It"). This allows you to make visual, auditory, and speech connections with its meaning.

- Identifying the type of word (Noun, verb, adverb, and adjective). Making this distinction helps you understand how to visualize the word. It helps you "chunk" the words into groups, and gives you clues on how to use the word.

- Place the word in context by using it in a sentence. Write this sentence down and read it aloud. This will give you an example of how the word is used.

- "Chunking". By breaking down the word list into groups of closely related words, you will learn them better and be able to remember them faster. Once you have group the terms, you can then make word clouds using a free online service. These word clouds provide visual cues to remembering the words and their meanings.

- Analogies. By creating analogies for essential words, you will be making connections that you can see on paper. These connections can trigger your memory and activate your ability to use the word in your writing as you begin to use them. Many of these analogies also use visual cues. In a sense, you can make a mental picture from the analogy.

- Mnemonics. A device such as a pattern of letters, ideas, or associations that assists in remembering something. A mnemonic is especially useful for remembering the order of a set of words or the order of a process.

- Morphology. The study of word roots, prefixes, and suffixes. By examining the structure of the words, you will gain insight into other words that are closely related, and learn how to best use the word.

- Visual metaphors. This is the most sophisticated and entertaining strategy for learning vocabulary. Create a "memory cartoon" using one or more of the vocabulary terms. This activity triggers the visual part of your memory and makes fast, permanent, imprints of the word on your memory. By combining the terms in your visual metaphor, you can "chunk" the entire set of vocabulary terms into several visual metaphors and benefit from the brain's tendency to group these terms.

The activities in this book are designed to imprint the words and their meanings in your memory in different ways. By completing each activity, you will gain the necessary exposures to the word to make it a permanent part of your vocabulary. Each activity uses a different part of your memory. The result is that you will be comfortable using these words and be able to tell the difference between closely related words. The activities include:

A. Crossword Puzzles and Word Searches- These are proven to increase test scores and improve comprehension. Students frequently report that they are fun and engaging, while requiring them to analyze the structure and meaning of the words.

B. Matching- This activity is effective because it forces you to differentiate between many closely related terms.

C. Multiple Choice- This classic question format lends itself to vocabulary study perfectly. Most exams are in this format because they are simple to make, easy to score, and are a reliable type of assessment. (Perfect for the Vocabulary Master!) One strategy to use with multiple choice questions that enhance their effectiveness is to cover the answer choices while you read the question. After reading the question, see if you can answer it before looking at the choices. Then look at the choices to see if you match one of them.

Conducting a thorough "word study" of your insider language will take time and effort, but the rewards will be well worth it. By following this guide and completing the exercises thoughtfully, you will become a stronger, more effective, and satisfied student. Best of luck on your mastery of this Insider Language!

Insider Language Strategies

"See It, Say It!" Reading your Insider Language set aloud

"IT IS BETTER TO FAIL IN ORIGINALITY THAN TO SUCCEED IN IMITATION."
–HERMAN MELVILLE

Reading aloud is the foundation for the development of an Insider Language. It is the single most important thing you can do for vocabulary acquisition. Done correctly, it engages the visual, auditory, and speech centers of the brain and hastens its storage in your long-term memory.

Reading aloud demonstrates the relationship between the printed word and its meaning.

You can read aloud on a higher level than you can initially understand, so reading aloud makes complex ideas more accessible and exposes you to vocabulary and patterns that are not part of your typical speech. Reading aloud helps you understand the complicated text better and makes more challenging text easier to grasp and understand. Reading aloud helps you to develop the "habits of mind" the strongest students use.

Reading aloud will make connections to concepts in the reading that requires you to relate the new vocabulary to things you already know. Go to the glossary at the end of this book and for each word complete the five steps outlined below:

1. Read the word and its definition aloud. Focus on the sound of the word and how it looks on the paper.
2. Read the word aloud again try to say three or four similar words; this will help you build connections to closely related words.
3. Read the word aloud a third time. Try to make a connection to something you have read or heard.
4. Visualize the concept described in the term. Paint a mental picture of the word in use.
5. Try to think of the opposite of the word. Discovering a close antonym will help you place this word in context.

Create a sentence using the word in its proper context

"OPPORTUNITIES DON'T HAPPEN. YOU CREATE THEM." –CHRIS GROSSER

Context means the circumstances that form the setting for an event, statement, or idea, and which it can be fully understood and assessed. Synonyms for context include conditions, factors, situation, background, and setting.

Place the word in context by using it in a sentence. Write this sentence down and read it aloud. By creating sentences, you are practicing using the word correctly. If you strive to make these sentences interesting and creative, they will become more memorable and effective in activating your long-term memory.

Identify the Parts of Speech
"SUCCESS IS NOT FINAL; FAILURE IS NOT FATAL: IT IS THE COURAGE TO CONTINUE THAT COUNTS." –WINSTON S. CHURCHILL

Read through each term in the glossary and make a note of what part of speech each term is. Studying and identifying parts of speech shows us how the words relate to each other. It also helps you create a visualization of each term. Below are brief descriptions of the parts of speech for you to use as a guide.

VERB: A word denoting action, occurrence, or existence. Examples: walk, hop, whisper, sweat, dribbles, feels, sleeps, drink, smile, are, is, was, has.

NOUN: A word that names a person, place, thing, idea, animal, quality, or action. Nouns are the subject of the sentence. Examples: dog, Tom, Florida, CD, pasta, hate, tiger.

ADJECTIVE: A word that modifies, qualifies, or describes nouns and pronouns. Generally, adjectives appear immediately before the words they modify. Examples: smart girl, gifted teacher, old car, red door.

ADVERB: A word that modifies verbs, adjectives and other adverbs. An "ly" ending almost always changes an adjective to an adverb. Examples: ran swiftly, worked slowly, and drifted aimlessly. Many adverbs do not end in "ly." However, all adverbs identify when, where, how, how far, how much, etc. Examples: run hot, lived hard, moved right, study smart.

Chunking

Chunking is when you take a set of words and break it down into groups based on a common relationship. Research has shown that our brains learn by chunking information. By grouping your terms, you will be able to recall large sets of these words easily. To help make your chunking go easily use an online word cloud generator to make a set of word clouds representing your chunks.

1. Study the glossary and decide how you want to chunk the set of words. You can group by part of speech, topic, letter of the alphabet, word length, etc. Try to find an easy way to group each term.
2. Once you have your different groups, visit www.wordclouds.com to create a custom word cloud for each group. Print each one of these clouds and post it in a prominent place to serve as constant visual aids for your learning.

Analogies

An analogy is a comparison in which an idea or a thing is compared to another thing that is quite different from it. Analogies aim at explaining an idea by comparing it to something that is familiar. Metaphors and similes are tools used to create analogies.

Analogies are useful for learning vocabulary because they require you to analyze a word (or words), and then transfer that analysis to another word. This transfer reinforces the understanding of all the words.

As you analyze the relationships between the analogies you are creating, you will begin to understand the complex relationships between the seemingly unrelated words.

_A_ is to _B_ as _C_ is to _D_

This can be written using colons in place of the terms "is to" and "as."

A:B::C:D

The two items on the left (items A & B) describe a relationship and are separated by a single colon. The two items on the right (items C & D) are shown on the right and are also separated by a colon. Together, both sides are then separated by two colons in the middle, as shown here: Tall: Short :: Skinny: Fat. The relationship used in this analogy is the antonym.

How to create an analogy

Start with the basic formula for an analogy:

_____ : _____ :: _____ : _____

Next, we will examine a simple synonym analogy:

<u>automobile</u> : <u>car</u> :: <u>box</u> : <u>crate</u>

The key to figuring out a set of word analogies is determining the relationship between the paired set of words.

Here is a list of the most common types of Analogies and examples

Synonym	Scream : Yell :: Push : Shove
Antonym	Rich : Poor :: Empty : Full
Cause is to Effect	Prosperity : Happiness :: Success : Joy
A Part is to its Whole	Toe : Foot :: Piece : Set
An Object to its Function	Car : Travel :: Read : Learn
A Item is to its Category	Tabby : House Cat :: Doberman : Dog
Word is a symptom of the other	Pain : Fracture :: Wheezing : Allergy
An object and it's description	Glass : Brittle :: Lead : Dense
The word is lacking the second word	Amputee : Limb :: Deaf : Hearing
The first word Hinders the second word	Shackles : Movement :: Stagger : Walk
The first word helps the action of the second	Knife : Bread :: Screwdriver : Screw
This word is made up of the second word	Sweater : Wool :: Jeans : Denim
A word and it's definition	Cede: Break Away :: Abolish : To get rid of

Using words from the glossary, make a set of analogies using each one. As a bonus, use more than one glossary term in a single analogy.

_____ : _____ :: _____ : _____

Name the relationship between the words in your analogy:_____

_____ : _____ :: _____ : _____

Name the relationship between the words in your analogy:_____

_____ : _____ :: _____ : _____

Name the relationship between the words in your analogy:_____

Mnemonics

"It isn't the mountains ahead to climb that wear you out; it's the pebble in your shoe." —Muhammad Ali

A mnemonic is a learning technique that helps you retain and remember information. Mnemonics are one of the best learning methods for remembering lists or processes in order. Mnemonics make the material more meaningful by adding associations and creating patterns. Interestingly, mnemonics may work better when they utilize absurd, startling, or shocking examples and references. Mnemonics help organize the information so that you can easily retrieve it later. By giving you associations and cues, mnemonics allow you to form a mental structure ordering a list or process to help you remember it better. This mental structure allows you to create a structure of association between items that may not appear to have any relationship. Mnemonics typically use references that are easy to visualize and thus easier to remember. Through visualization of vivid images and references, the information is much easier to imprint into long-term memory. The power of making mnemonics lies in converting dull, inert and uninspiring information into something vibrant and memorable.

How to make simple and effective mnemonics
Some of the best mnemonics help us remember simple rules or lists in order.

Step 1. Take a list of terms you are trying to remember in order. For example, we will use the scientific method:

observation, question, hypothesis, methods, results, and conclusion.

Next, we will replace each word on the list with a new word that starts with the same letter. These new words will together form a vivid sentence that is easy to remember:

Objectionable Queens Haunted Macho Rednecks Creatively.

As silly as the above sentence seems, it is easy to remember, and now we can call on this sentence to remind us of the order of the scientific method.

Visit http://www.mnemonicgenerator.com/ and try typing in a list of words. It is fun to see the mnemonics that it makes and shows how easy it is to make great mnemonics to help your studying.

Using vivid words in your mnemonics allows you to see the sentence you are making. Words that are gross, scary, or name interesting animals are helpful. Profanity is also useful because the shock value can trigger memory. The following are lists of vivid words to use in your mnemonics:

Gross words
Moist, Gurgle, Phlegm, Fetus, Curd, Smear, Squirt, Chunky, Orifice, Maggots, Viscous, Queasy, Bulbous, Pustule, Putrid, Fester, Secrete, Munch, Vomit, Ooze, Dripping, Roaches, Mucus, Stink, Stank, Stunk, Slurp, Pus, Lick, Salty, Tongue, Fart, Flatulence, Hemorrhoid.

Interesting Animals
Aardvark, Baboon, Chicken, Chinchilla, Duck, Dragonfly, Emu, Electric Eel, Frog, Flamingo, Gecko, Hedgehog, Hyena, Iguana, Jackal, Jaguar, Leopard, Lynx, Minnow, Manatee, Mongoose, Neanderthal, Newt, Octopus, Oyster, Pelican, Penguin, Platypus, Quail, Racoon, Rattlesnake, Rhinoceros, Scorpion, Seahorse, Toucan, Turkey, Vulture, Weasel, Woodpecker, Yak, Zebra.

Superhero Words
Diabolical, Activate, Boom, Clutch, Dastardly, Dynamic, Dynamite, Shazam, Kaboom, Zip, Zap, Zoom, Zany, Crushing, Smashing, Exploding, Ripping, Tearing.

Scary Words
Apparition, Bat, Chill, Demon, Eerie, Fangs, Genie, Hell, Lantern, Macabre, Nightmare, Owl, Ogre, Phantasm, Repulsive, Scarecrow, Tarantula, Undead, Vampire, Wraith, Zombie.

There are several types of mnemonics that can help your memory.

1. Images
Visual mnemonics are a type of **mnemonic** that works by associating an image with characters or objects whose name sounds like the item that must be memorized. This is one of the easiest ways to create effective mnemonics. An example would be to use the shape of numbers to help memorize a long list of them. Numbers can be memorized by their shapes, so that: 0 -looks like an egg; 1 -a pencil, or a candle; 2 -a snake; 3 -an ear; 4 -a sailboat; 5 -a key; 6 -a comet; 7 -a knee; 8 -a snowman; 9 -a comma.

Another type of visual mnemonic is the word-length mnemonic in which the number of letters in each word corresponds to a digit. This simple mnemonic gives pi to seven decimal places:

3.141582 becomes "How I wish I could calculate pi."

Of course, you could use this type of mnemonic to create a longer sentence showing the digits of an important number. Some people have used this type of mnemonic to memorize thousands of digits.

Using the hands is also an important tool for creating visual objects. Making the hands into specific shapes can help us remember the pattern of things or the order of a list of things.

2. Rhyming

Rhyming mnemonics are quick ways to make things memorable. A classic example is a mnemonic for the number of days in each month:
"30 days hath September, April, June, and November.
All the rest have 31
Except February, my dear son.
It has 28, and that is fine
But in Leap Year it has 29."

Another example of a rhyming mnemonic is a common spelling rule:
"I before e except after c
or when sounding like a
in neighbor and weigh."

Use **rhymer.com** to get large lists of rhyming words.

3. Homonym

A homonym is one of a group of words that share the same pronunciation but have different meanings, whether spelled the same or not.

Try saying what you're attempting to remember out loud or very quickly, and see if anything leaps out. If you know other languages, using similar-sounding words from those can be effective.

You could also browse this list of homonyms
at http://www.cooper.com/alan/homonym_list.html.

4. Onomatopoeia

An Onomatopeia is a word that phonetically imitates, resembles or suggests the source of the sound that it describes. Are there any noises made by the thing you're trying to memorize? Is it often associated with some other sound? Failing that, just make up a noise that seems to fit.

Achoo, ahem, baa, bam, bark, beep, beep beep, belch, bleat, boo, boo hoo, boom, burp, buzz, chirp, click clack, crash, croak, crunch, cuckoo, dash, drip, ding dong, eek, fizz, flit, flutter, gasp, grrr, ha ha, hee hee, hiccup, hiss, hissing, honk, icky, itchy, jiggly, jangle, knock knock, lush, la la la, mash, meow, moan, murmur, neigh, oink, ouch, plop, pow, quack, quick, rapping, rattle, ribbit, roar, rumble, rustle, scratch, sizzle, skittering, snap crackle pop, splash, splish splash, spurt, swish, swoosh, tap, tapping, tick tock, tinkle, tweet, ugh, vroom, wham, whinny, whip, whooping, woof.

5. Acronyms

An acronym is a word or name formed as an abbreviation from the initial components of a word, such as NATO, which stands for North Atlantic Treaty Organization. If you're trying to memorize something involving letters, this is often a good bet. A lot of famous mnemonics are acronyms, such as ROYGBIV which stands for the order of colors in the light spectrum (Red, Orange, Yellow, Green, Blue, Indigo, and Violet).
A great acronym generator to try is: www.all-acronyms.com.

A different spin on an acronym is a backronym. A **backronym** is a specially constructed phrase that is supposed to be the source of a word that is an acronym. A backronym is constructed by creating a new phrase to fit an already existing word, name, or acronym.

The word is a combination of *backward* and *acronym*, and has been defined as a "reverse acronym." For example, the United States Department of Justice assigns to their Amber Alert program the meaning "**A**merica's **M**issing: **B**roadcast **E**mergency **R**esponse." The process can go either way to make good mnemonics.

Visit: https://arthurdick.com/projects/backronym/ to try out a simple backronym generator.

6. Anagrams

An anagram is a direct word switch or word play, the result of rearranging the letters of a word or phrase to produce a new word or phrase, using all the original letters exactly once; for example, the word anagram can be rearranged into nag-a-ram.

Try re-arranging letters or components and see if anything memorable emerges. Visit http://www.nameacronym.net/ to use a simple anagram generator.

One particularly memorable form of anagram is the spoonerism, where you swap the initial syllables or letters of words to make new phrases. These are usually humorous, and this makes them easier to remember. Here are some examples:

"Is it kisstomary to cuss the bride?" (as opposed to "customary to kiss")
"The Lord is a shoving leopard." (instead of "a loving shepherd")
"A blushing crow." ("crushing blow")
"A well-boiled icicle" ("well-oiled bicycle")
"You were fighting a liar in the quadrangle." ("lighting a fire")
"Is the bean dizzy?" (as opposed to "is the dean busy?")

7. Stories

Make up quick stories or incidents involving the material you want to memorize. For larger chunks of information, the stories can get more elaborate. Structured stories are particularly good for remembering lists or other sequenced information. Have a look at https://en.wikipedia.org/wiki/Method_of_loci for a more advanced memory sequencing technique.

Visual Metaphors

"LIMITS, LIKE FEAR, IS OFTEN AN ILLUSION." –MICHAEL JORDAN

What is a Metaphor?

A metaphor is a figure of speech that refers to one thing by mentioning another thing. Metaphors provide clarity and identify hidden similarities between two seemingly unrelated ideas. A visual metaphor is an image that creates a link between different ideas.

Visual metaphors help us use our understanding of the world to learn new concepts, skills, and ideas. Visual metaphors help us relate new material to what we already know. Visual metaphors must be clear and simple enough to spark a connection and understanding. Visual metaphors should use familiar things to help you be less fearful of new, complex, or challenging topics. Metaphors trigger a sense of familiarity so that you are more accepting of the new idea. Metaphors work best when you associate a familiar, easy to understand idea with a challenging, obscure, or abstract concept.

How to make a visual metaphor

1. Brainstorm using the words of the concept. Use different fonts, colors, or shapes to represent parts of the concept.

2. Merge these images together

3. Show the process using arrows, accents, etc.

4. Think about the story line your metaphor projects.

Examples of visual metaphors:

A skeleton used to show a framework of something.

A cloud showing an outline.

A bodybuilder whose muscles represent supporting ideas and details.

A sandwich where the meat, tomato, and lettuce represent supporting ideas.

A recipe card to show a process.

Your metaphor should be accurate. It should be complex enough to convey meaning, but simple and clear enough to be easily understood.

Morphology
"SCIENCE IS THE CAPTAIN, AND PRACTICE THE SOLDIERS." LEONARDO DA VINCI

Morphology is the study of the origin, roots, suffixes, and prefixes of the words. Understanding the meaning of prefixes, suffixes, and roots make it easier to decode the meaning of new vocabulary. Having the ability to decode using morphology increases text comprehension when initially reading as well.

The capability of identifying meaningful parts of words (morphemes), including prefixes, suffixes, and roots can be helpful. Identifying morphemes improves decoding accuracy and fluency. Reading speed improves when you can decode larger chunks of text quickly. When you can recognize morphemes in words, you will be better able to make sense of new words in context. Below are charts containing the most common prefixes, suffixes, and root words. Use them to help you decode your vocabulary terms.

Prefixes

Prefix	Meaning	Example words and meanings	
a, ab, abs	away from	absent abdicate	not to be present, to give up an office or throne.
ad, a, ac, af, ag, an, ar, at, as	to, toward	Advance advantage	To move forward To have the upper hand
anti	against	Antidote antisocial antibiotic	To repair poisoning refers to someone who's not social
bi, bis	two	bicycle binary biweekly	two-wheeled cycle two number system every two weeks
circum, cir	around	circumnavigate circle	Travel around the world a figure that goes all around
com, con, co, col	with, together	Complete Complement	To finish To go along with
de	away from, down, the opposite of	depart detour	to go away from to go out of your way
dis, dif, di	apart	dislike dishonest distant	not to like not honest away
En-, em-	Cause to	Entrance	the way in.
epi	upon, on top of	epitaph epilogue epidemic	writing upon a tombstone speech at the end, on top of the rest
equ, equi	equal	equalize equitable	to make equal fair, equal
ex, e, ef	out, from	exit eject exhale	to go out to throw out to breathe out
Fore-	Before	Forewarned	To have prior warning

Prefix	Meaning	Example Words and Meanings	
in, il, ir, im, en	in, into	Infield Imbibe	The inner playing field to take part in
in, il, ig, ir, im	not	inactive ignorant irreversible irritate	not active not knowing not reversible to put into discomfort
inter	between, among	international interact	among nations to mix with
mal, male	bad, ill, wrong	malpractice malfunction	bad practice fail to function, bad function
Mid	Middle	Amidships	In the middle of a ship
mis	wrong, badly	misnomer	The wrong name
mono	one, alone, single	monocle	one lensed glasses
non	not, the reverse of	nonprofit	not making a profit
ob	in front, against, in front of, in the way of	Obsolete	No longer needed
omni	everywhere, all	omnipresent omnipotent	always present, everywhere all powerful
Over	On top	Overdose	Take too much medication
Pre	Before	Preview	Happens before a show.
per	through	Permeable pervasive	to pass through, all encompassing
poly	many	Polygamy polygon	many spouses figure with many sides
post	after	postpone postmortem	to do after after death
pre	before, earlier than	Predict Preview	To know before To view before release
pro	forward, going ahead of, supporting	proceed pro-war promote	to go forward supporting the war to raise or move forward
re	again, back	retell recall reverse	to tell again to call back to go back
se	apart	secede seclude	to withdraw, become apart to stay apart from others
Semi	Half	Semipermeable	Half-permeable

Prefix	Meaning	Example Words and Meanings	
Sub	under, less than	Submarine	under water
super	over, above, greater	superstar superimpose	a start greater than her stars to put over something else
trans	across	transcontinental transverse	across the continent to lie or go across
un, uni	one	unidirectional unanimous unilateral	having one direction sharing one view having one side
un	not	uninterested unhelpful unethical	not interested not helpful not ethical

Roots

Root	Meaning	Example words & meanings	
act, ag	to do, to act	Agent Activity	One who acts as a representative Action
Aqua	Water	Aquamarine	The color of water
Aud	To hear	Auditorium	A place to hear music
apert	open	Aperture	An opening
bas	low	Basement Basement	Something that is low, at the bottom A room that is low
Bio	Living thing	Biological	Living matter
cap, capt, cip, cept, ceive	to take, to hold, to seize	Captive Receive Capable Recipient	One who is held To take Able to take hold of things One who takes hold or receives
ced, cede, ceed, cess	to go, to give in	Precede Access Proceed	To go before Means of going to To go forward
Cogn	Know	Cognitive	Ability to think
cred, credit	to believe	Credible Incredible Credit	Believable Not believable Belief, trust
curr, curs, cours	to run	Current Precursory Recourse	Now in progress, running Running (going) before To run for aid
Cycle	Circle	Lifecycle	The circle of life
dic, dict	to say	Dictionary Indict	A book explaining words (sayings)

Root	Meaning	Examples and meanings	
duc, duct	to lead	Induce	To lead to action
		Conduct	To lead or guide
		Aqueduct	Pipe that leads water somewhere
equ	equal, even	Equality	Equal in social, political rights
		Equanimity	Evenness of mind, tranquility
fac, fact, fic, fect, fy	to make, to do	Facile	Easy to do
		Fiction	Something that is made up
		Factory	Place that makes things
		Affect	To make a change in
fer, ferr	to carry, bring	Defer	To carry away
		Referral	Bring a source for help/information
Gen	Birth	Generate	To create something
graph	write	Monograph	A writing on a particular subject
		Graphite	A form of carbon used for writing
Loc	Place	Location	A place
Mater	Mother	Maternity	Expecting birth
Mem	Recall	Memory	The recall experiences
mit, mis	to send	Admit	To send in
		Missile	Something sent through the air
Nat	Born	Native	Born in a place
par	equal	Parity	Equality
		Disparate	No equal, not alike
Ped	Foot	Podiatrist	Foot doctor
Photo	Light	Photograph	A picture
plic	to fold, to bend, to turn	Complicate	To fold (mix) together
		Implicate	To fold in, to involve
pon, pos, posit, pose	to place	Component	A part placed together with others
		Transpose	A place across
		Compose	To put many parts into place
		Deposit	To place for safekeeping
scrib, script	to write	Describe	To write about or tell about
		Transcript	A written copy
		Subscription	A written signature or document
sequ, secu	to follow	Sequence	In following order

Root	Meaning	Examples and Meanings	
Sign	Mark	Signal	to alert somebody
spec, spect, spic	to appear, to look, to see	Specimen Aspect	An example to look at One way to see something
sta, stat, sist,	to stand, or make stand	Constant	Standing with
stit, sisto	Stable, steady	Status Stable Desist	Social standing Steady (standing) To stand away from
Struct	To build	Construction	To build a thing
tact	to touch	Contact Tactile	To touch together To be able to be touched
ten, tent, tain	to hold	Tenable Retentive Maintain	Able to be held, holding Holding To keep or hold up
tend, tens, tent	to stretch	Extend Tension	To stretch or draw out Stretched
Therm	Temperature	Thermometer	Detects temperature
tract	to draw	Attract Contract	To draw together An agreement drawn up
ven, vent	to come	Convene Advent	To come together A coming
Vis	See	Invisible	Cannot be seen
ver, vert, vers	to turn	Avert Revert Reverse	To turn away To turn back To turn around

Crossword Puzzles

1. *Using the Across and Down clues, write the correct words in the numbered grid below.*

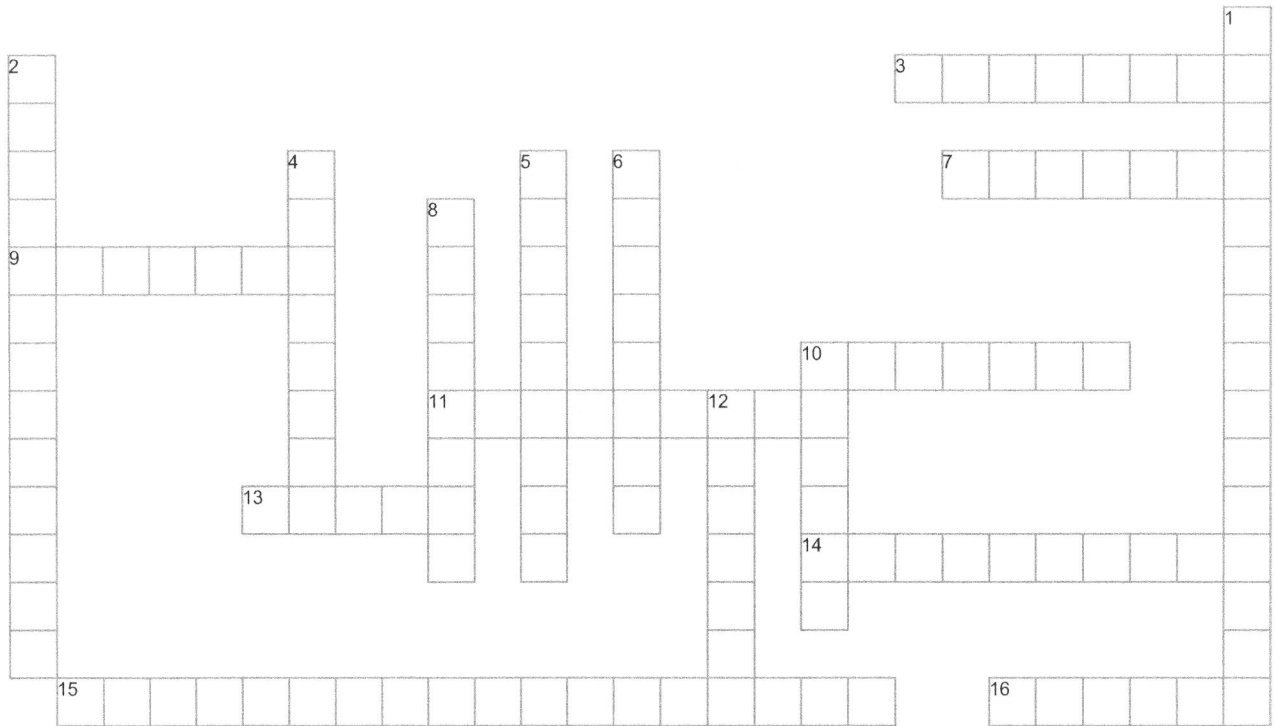

ACROSS

3. Judge; consider.
7. Guess; tell what will happen next.
9. Use details from the text to explain your response.
10. A simplified drawing.
11. To come up with.
13. To produce words.
14. To draw or make pictures to explain.
15. A sentence that pulls together or summarizes the main idea and provides a definite ending point for a paragraph or written piece.
16. Make out; break apart.

DOWN

1. Text that the author presents as an argument.
2. The way a text is presented: introduction, headings and
4. A comparison of two unlike things by describing one is the other.
5. To make a product.
6. The way someone feels about something.
8. A word, phrase or clause used to describe or qualify another word, phrase or clause.
10. A single piece of information or fact about something.
12. Break apart; study the pieces.

A. Textual evidence
B. Attitude
C. Modifier
D. Analyze
E. Predict
F. Evaluate
G. Illustrate
H. Write
I. Support
J. Detail
K. Decode
L. Diagram
M. Text structure
N. Construct
O. Concluding sentence
P. Metaphor
Q. Formulate

2. *Using the Across and Down clues, write the correct words in the numbered grid below.*

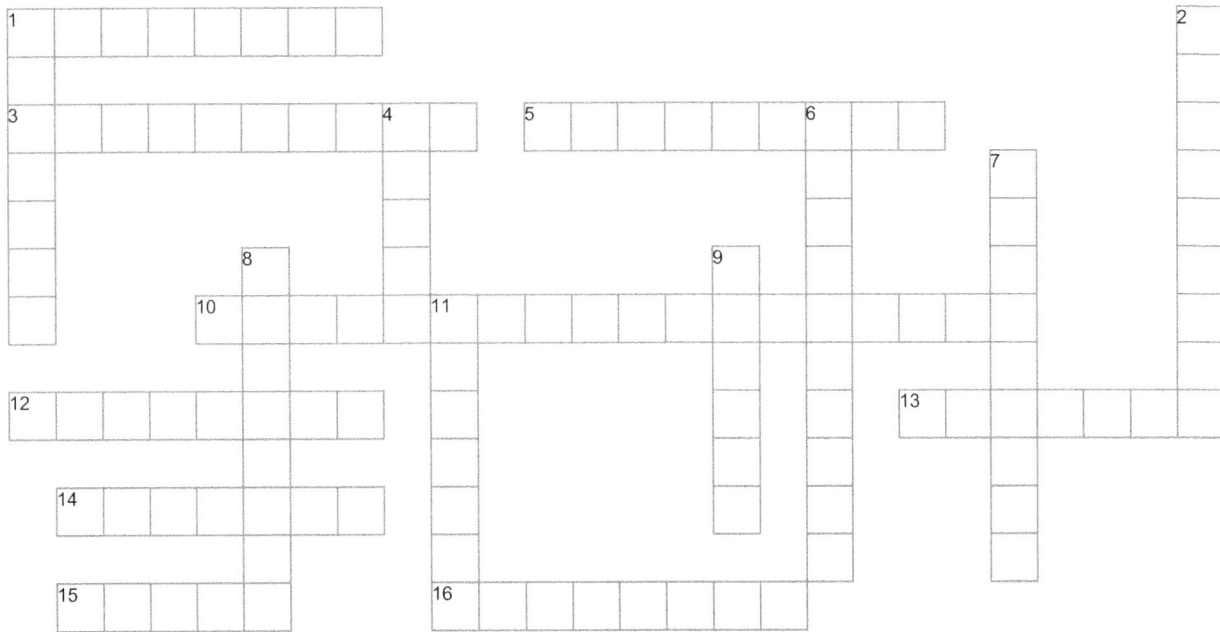

ACROSS

1. Order in which events, movements, or things follow each other.
3. Will probably happen; probably.
5. To think about carefully and form an opinion.
10. A sentence that pulls together or summarizes the main idea and provides a definite ending point for a paragraph or written piece.
12. A person who tells something; storyteller.
13. Exact or specific.
14. Using few words to give the most important information about something or a complete but brief account of things previously stated.
15. Anything that happens, especially something important or unusual.
16. Judge; consider.

DOWN

1. A short way of saying what the reading passage is about.
2. Copy; repeat.
4. Name; identify.
6. The basic definition or dictionary meaning of a word.
7. A conclusion reached based on reasoning and the use of given facts; a prediction.
8. To find differences.
9. Repeat; say again.
11. Use something to help find a solution.

A. Summary	B. Contrast	C. Evaluate	D. Label
E. Most likely	F. Retell	G. Concludes	H. Summary
I. Denotation	J. Precise	K. Reproduce	L. Event
M. Sequence	N. Utilize	O. Narrator	P. Concluding sentence
Q. Inference			

3. *Using the Across and Down clues, write the correct words in the numbered grid below.*

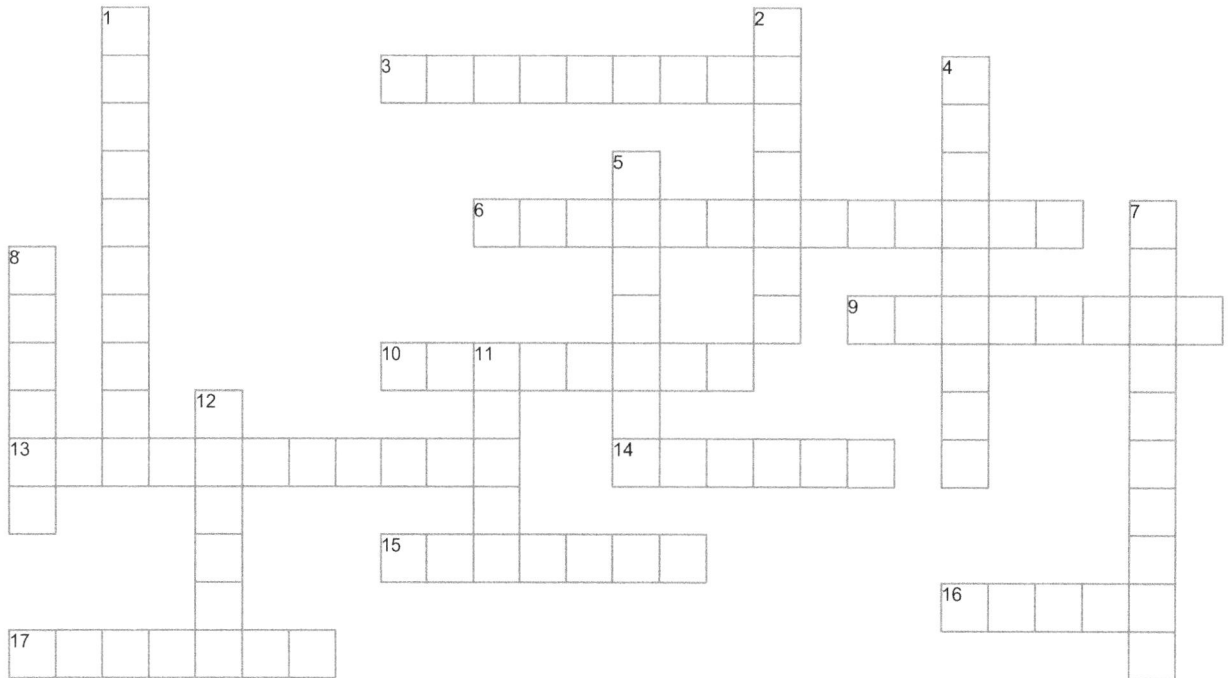

ACROSS

3. To determine the meaning of.
6. A punctuation mark ", " or ',' used at the beginning and ending of text that has been stated from a source.
9. Able to trust.
10. To tell or write about something in detail.
13. The main point of the story or the text; the unifying element of a story or text, sometimes called main idea or theme.
14. To choose.
15. Exact or specific.
16. Plain; rough copy.
17. To gather together.

DOWN

1. The ending, answer, or conclusion to a problem or story.
2. Use something to help find a solution.
4. To show to be true, to prove.
5. A style of print where the letters slope to the right; may be used to emphasize or to indicate the title of published work.
7. To draw or make pictures to explain.
8. To cause changes.
11. Say; affirm.
12. To make a product.

A. Illustrate   B. Precise   C. Utilize   D. State
E. Resolution   F. Reliable   G. Collect   H. Select
I. Describe   J. Italics   K. Draft   L. Central idea
M. Impact   N. Establish   O. Interpret   P. Create
Q. Quotation mark

4. *Using the Across and Down clues, write the correct words in the numbered grid below.*

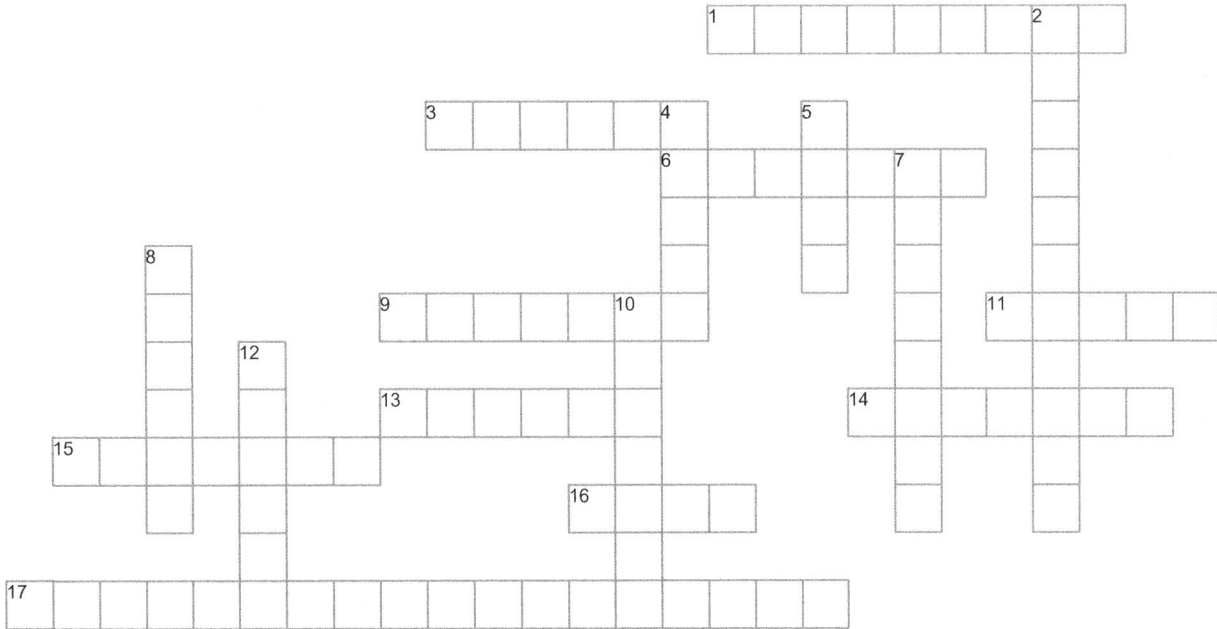

ACROSS

1. Copy; repeat.
3. To choose.
6. Think about; wonder about.
9. The reason someone does something.
11. Name; identify.
13. Give an answer; consequence.
14. An explanation for a picture or illustration.
15. Part; section.
16. To use a quote from the text to support an idea.
17. Words or expression different from literal language, changed or altered to make a linguistic point.

DOWN

2. All the meanings, associations, emotions, or tones that a word suggests.
4. Outline; map out.
5. The events that make up the story or the main part of the story. The events relate to each other in a pattern or sequence.
7. To find differences.
8. Change; alter.
10. The period and-or location in which a story takes place.
12. A group of lines in a poem (similar to a paragraph).

A. Result
B. Contrast
C. Stanza
D. Setting
E. Select
F. Reproduce
G. Reflect
H. Revise
I. Connotation
J. Passage
K. Plot
L. Cite
M. Trace
N. Label
O. Figurative language
P. Purpose
Q. Caption

5. *Using the Across and Down clues, write the correct words in the numbered grid below.*

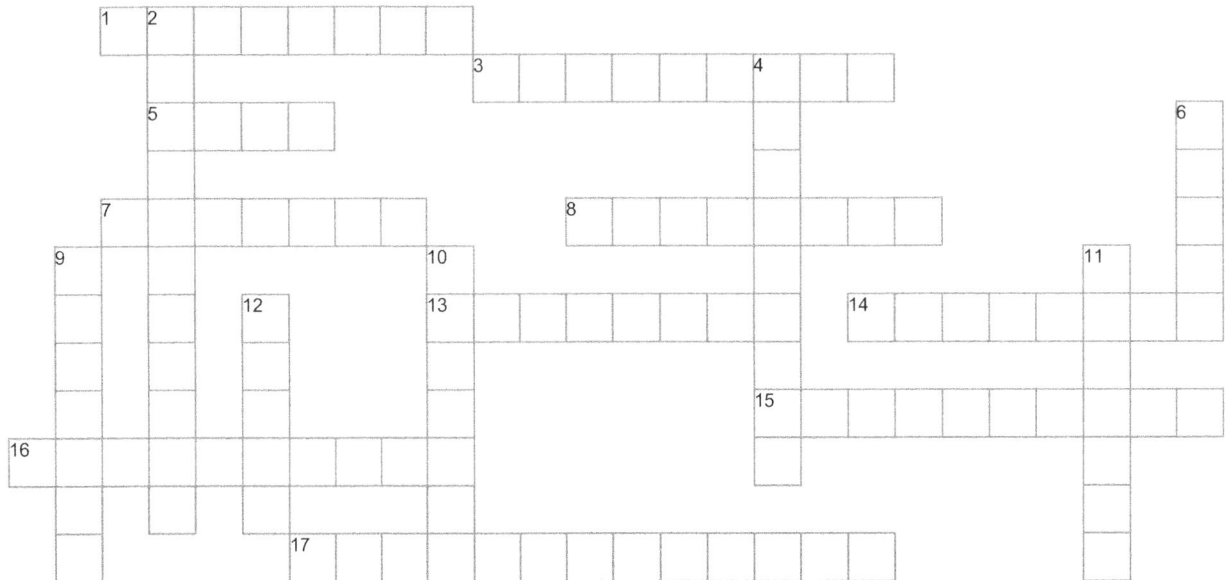

ACROSS

1. Name; label.
3. Sum it up; give a short version.
5. A temporary state of mind or feeling.
7. Break apart; study the pieces.
8. Not sure what is going to happen, waiting.
13. To judge or determine the quality or amount of something.
14. Able to trust.
15. To do something the same constantly.
16. To help happen or help cause.
17. A punctuation mark ", " or ',' used at the beginning and ending of text that has been stated from a source.

DOWN

2. Show; make plain.
4. To come up with a conclusion without valid evidence to support it.
6. Say; affirm.
9. To provide proof or evidence for.
10. Think about; wonder about.
11. Watch; notice.
12. To state a position or declare that something is true or factual, noun-a statement of truth or fact, typically pertaining to an idea that is disputed.

A. Reliable
B. Consistent
C. Inference
D. Identify
E. Mood
F. State
G. Quotation mark
H. Support
I. Evaluate
J. Reflect
K. Observe
L. Analyze
M. Contribute
N. Suspense
O. Summarize
P. Claim
Q. Demonstrate

6. *Using the Across and Down clues, write the correct words in the numbered grid below.*

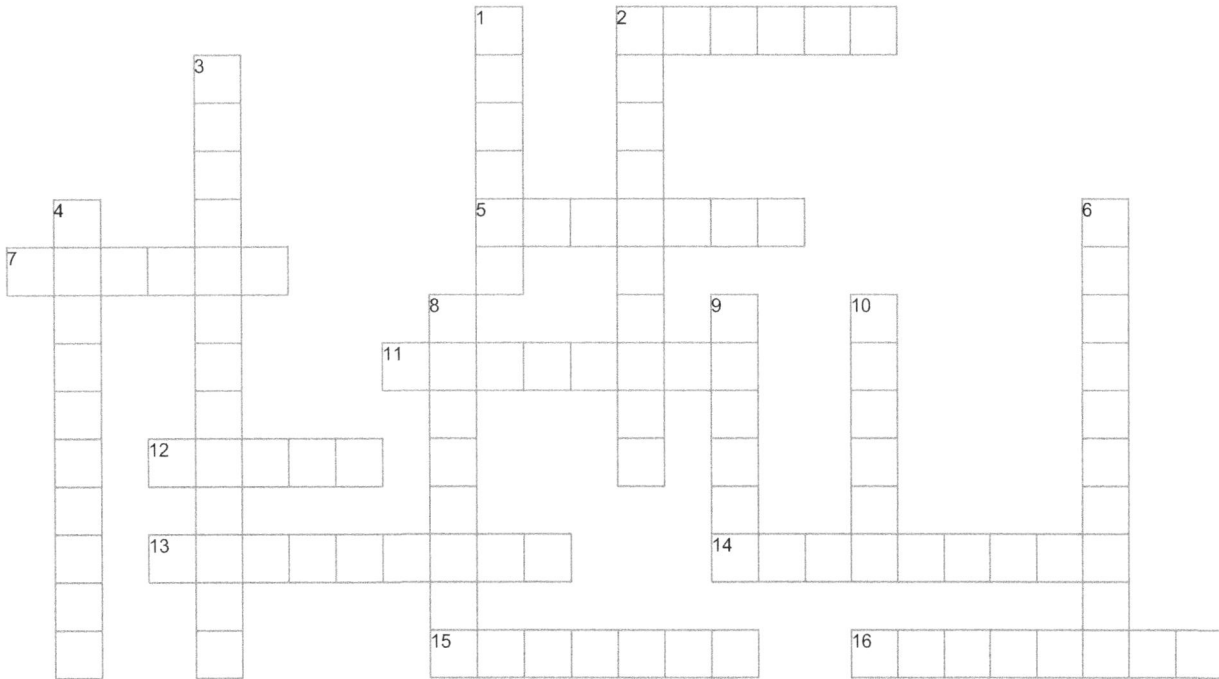

ACROSS

2. Give an answer; consequence.
5. To give details to make something clear.
7. To show or make known.
11. Tell about; explain.
12. To explain an idea or make a conclusion by looking closely at evidence in text.
13. A story.
14. Able to do its job to the best ability.
15. A part of a reading passage.
16. A person who tells something; storyteller.

DOWN

1. To make things or ideas known to others; to share or to get ideas across to others.
2. The ending, answer, or conclusion to a problem or story.
3. A punctuation mark ", " or ',' used at the beginning and ending of text that has been stated from a source.
4. The basic definition or dictionary meaning of a word.
6. To do something the same constantly.
8. To tell or write about something in detail.
9. Describe; characterize.
10. Make out; break apart.

A. Decode
B. Narrator
C. Result
D. Resolution
E. Define
F. Consistent
G. Excerpt
H. Describe
I. Infer
J. Reveal
K. Denotation
L. Explain
M. Quotation mark
N. Convey
O. Narrative
P. Describe
Q. Effective

7. *Using the Across and Down clues, write the correct words in the numbered grid below.*

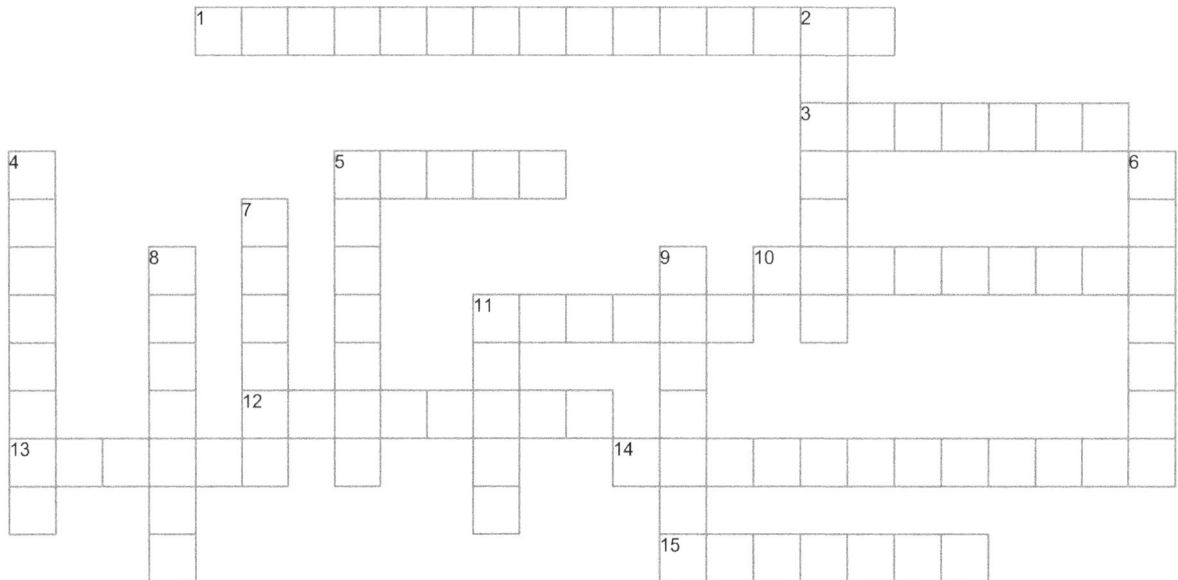

ACROSS

1. Text that the author presents as an argument.
3. To think of what will happen in the future or later.
5. Anything that happens, especially something important or unusual.
10. To think about carefully and form an opinion.
11. To make things or ideas known to others; to share or to get ideas across to others.
12. Explain how things are different.
13. Describe; characterize.
14. A part of the story that is important.
15. Give the facts; back up with details.

DOWN

2. An explanation for a picture or illustration.
4. to decide based upon information stated in the reading passages.
5. Look at; inspect.
6. A usually short piece of written work that focuses on a topic.
7. A book, person, or document used to provide information or data.
8. Guess; tell what will happen next.
9. Provide exact items; be specific.
11. To state a position or declare that something is true or factual, noun-a statement of truth or fact, typically pertaining to an idea that is disputed.

A. Event
E. Details
I. Predict
M. Concludes
Q. Passage

B. Source
F. Contrast
J. Support
N. Examine

C. Significance
G. Textual evidence
K. Conclude
O. Predict

D. Claim
H. Convey
L. Caption
P. Define

8. *Using the Across and Down clues, write the correct words in the numbered grid below.*

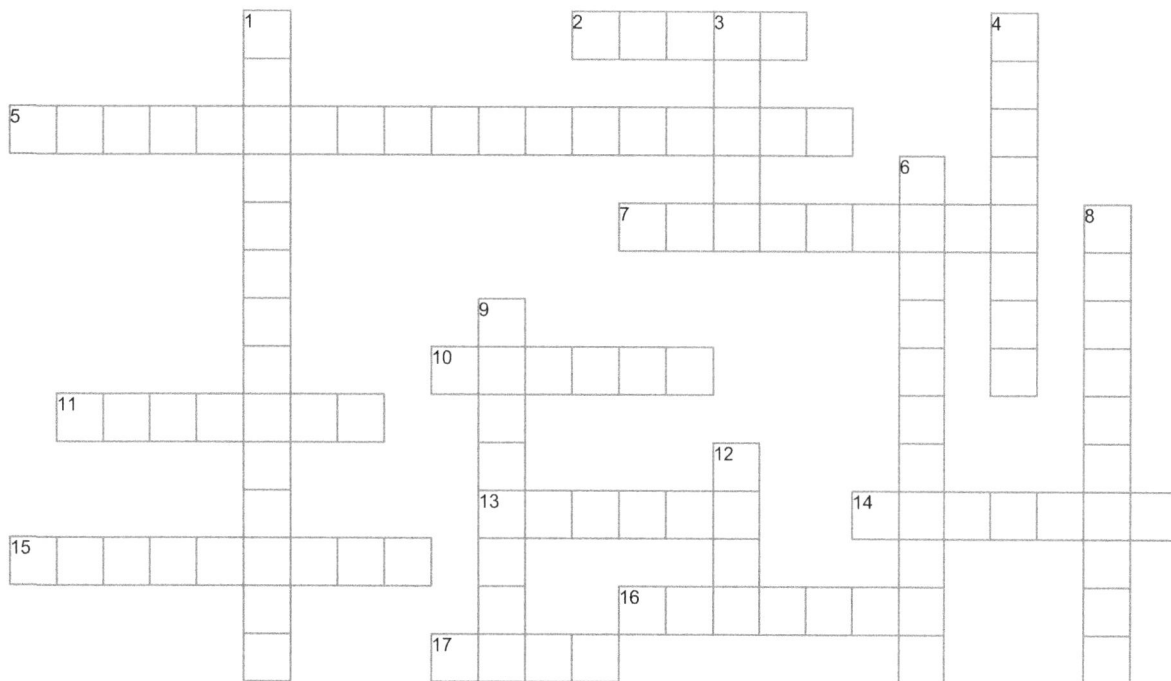

ACROSS

2. To produce words.
5. Words that may not literally mean what they say.
7. A way of looking or thinking about something.
10. Repeat; say again.
11. Use details from the text to explain your response.
13. Change; alter.
14. A short way of saying what the reading passage is about.
15. To come up with a conclusion without valid evidence to support it.
16. Provide exact items; be specific.
17. A book or other written work or printed work.

DOWN

1. Read and examine text in detail looking for important ideas.
3. Outline; map out.
4. Job, what it does.
6. To tell as different.
8. A restatement of the meaning of a text or passage using other words.
9. Tell about; explain.
12. The reading passage.

A. Trace
B. Revise
C. Text
D. Retell
E. Distinguish
F. Support
G. Text
H. Function
I. Analysis of text
J. Summary
K. Details
L. Describe
M. Write
N. Figurative language
O. Paraphrase
P. Inference
Q. Viewpoint

9. *Using the Across and Down clues, write the correct words in the numbered grid below.*

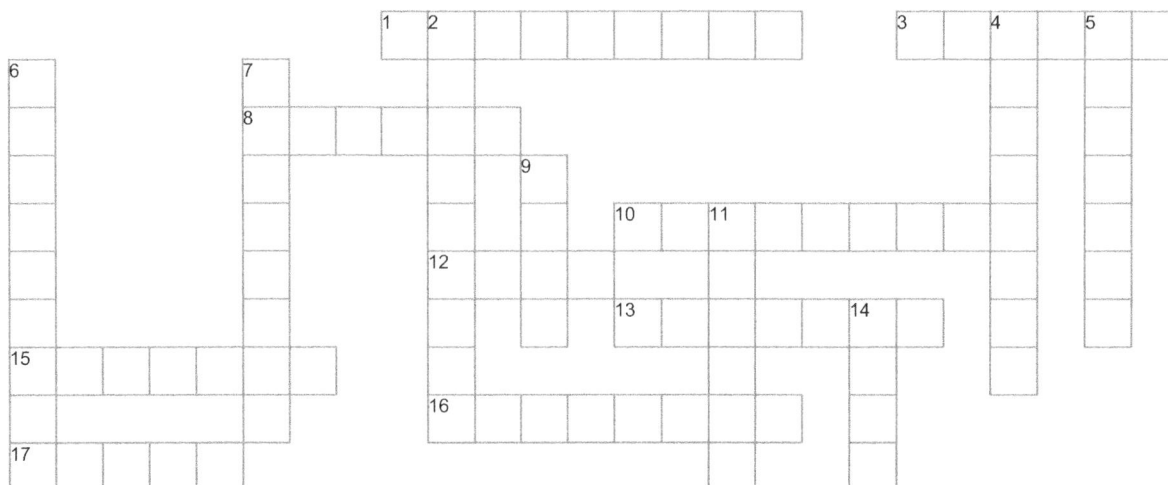

ACROSS

1. Explain the meaning; make clear.
3. Judge; consider.
8. To put down in writing so that it is saved.
10. Imagine; think about.
12. A book or other written work or printed work.
13. To gather together.
15. To look at text carefully by paying attention to its parts, its words, its figurative language, and its tone.
16. Proof; information in the text that proves a point.
17. Name; identify.

DOWN

2. A story.
4. Not sure what is going to happen, waiting.
5. Give the facts; back up with details.
6. Helps to support the central idea in an important way. Authors elaborate using examples or anecdotes.
7. Put in order; arrange.
9. The reading passage.
11. To choose.
14. To use a quote from the text to support an idea.

A. Suspense   B. Record   C. Analyze   D. Visualize   E. Interpret   F. Text
G. Collect   H. Assess   I. Organize J. Label   K. Evidence   L. Text
M. Select   N. Key detail O. Narrative P. Cite   Q. Support

10. *Using the Across and Down clues, write the correct words in the numbered grid below.*

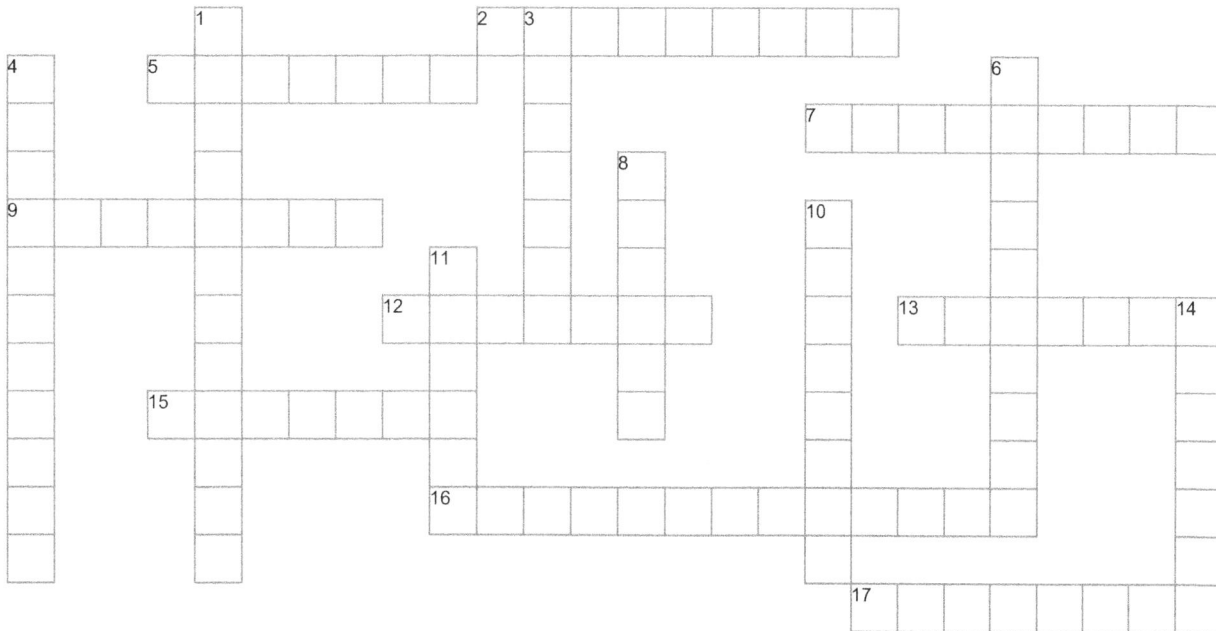

ACROSS

2. A story.
5. To consider an idea.
7. Helps to support the central idea in an important way. Authors elaborate using examples or anecdotes.
9. Stated clearly and in detail.
12. To work out, grow, or expand.
13. A style of print where the letters slope to the right; may be used to emphasize or to indicate the title of published work.
15. Part; section.
16. The way a text is presented: introduction, headings and
17. Explain how things are different.

DOWN

1. A part of the story that is important.
3. Break apart; study the pieces.
4. To search for an answer to a solution.
6. to make a statement based upon details from the reading passage that might be true in other situations.
8. Make out; break apart.
10. Proof; information in the text that proves a point.
11. To choose.
14. Give the facts; back up with details.

A. Explicit   B. Evidence   C. Significance   D. Key detail   E. Generalize
F. Contrast   G. Italics   H. Discuss   I. Select   J. Narrative
K. Analyze   L. Text structure   M. Develop   N. Decode   O. Passage
P. Support   Q. Investigate

11. *Using the Across and Down clues, write the correct words in the numbered grid below.*

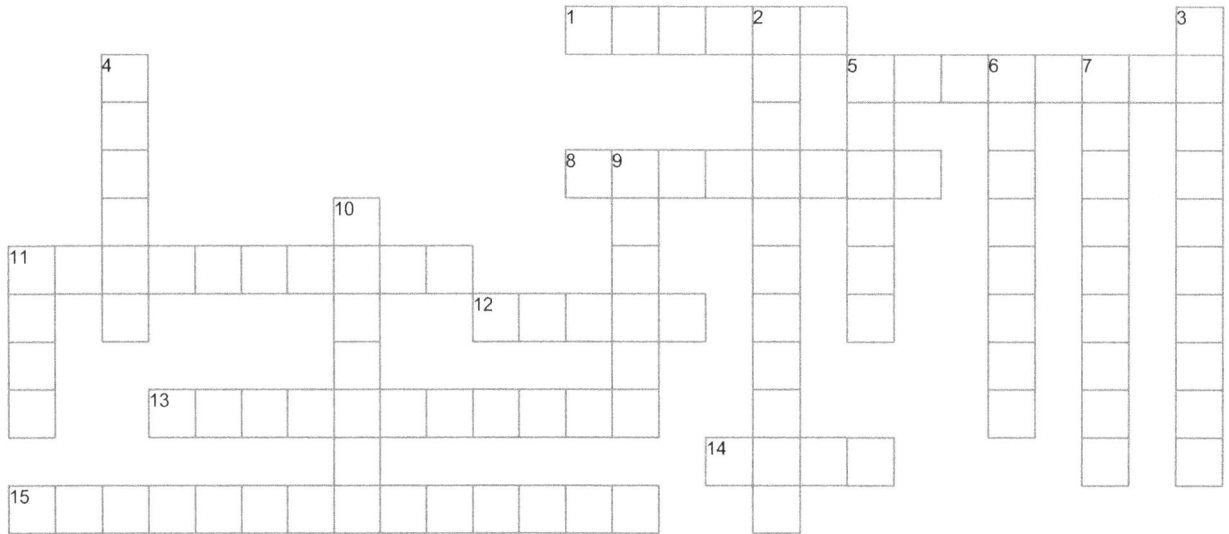

ACROSS

1. To choose.
5. To tell the facts, details.
8. To recognize or establish as being a person or thing.
11. Will probably happen; probably.
12. To state a position or declare that something is true or factual, noun-a statement of truth or fact, typically pertaining to an idea that is disputed.
13. Data that is based on numbers.
14. Above all others, most desirable.
15. Read and examine text in detail looking for important ideas.

DOWN

2. The main point of the story or the text; the unifying element of a story or text, sometimes called main idea or theme.
3. The ending, answer, or conclusion to a problem or story.
4. Judge; consider.
5. Support; uphold.
6. Put in order; sort.
7. To come up with a conclusion without valid evidence to support it.
9. Describe; characterize.
10. Provide exact items; be specific.
11. A temporary state of mind or feeling.

A. Details   B. Resolution   C. Analysis of text   D. Central idea
E. Claim   F. Mood   G. Define   H. Assess
I. Most likely   J. Select   K. Inference   L. Qualitative
M. Classify   N. Best   O. Identify   P. Describe
Q. Defend

12. *Using the Across and Down clues, write the correct words in the numbered grid below.*

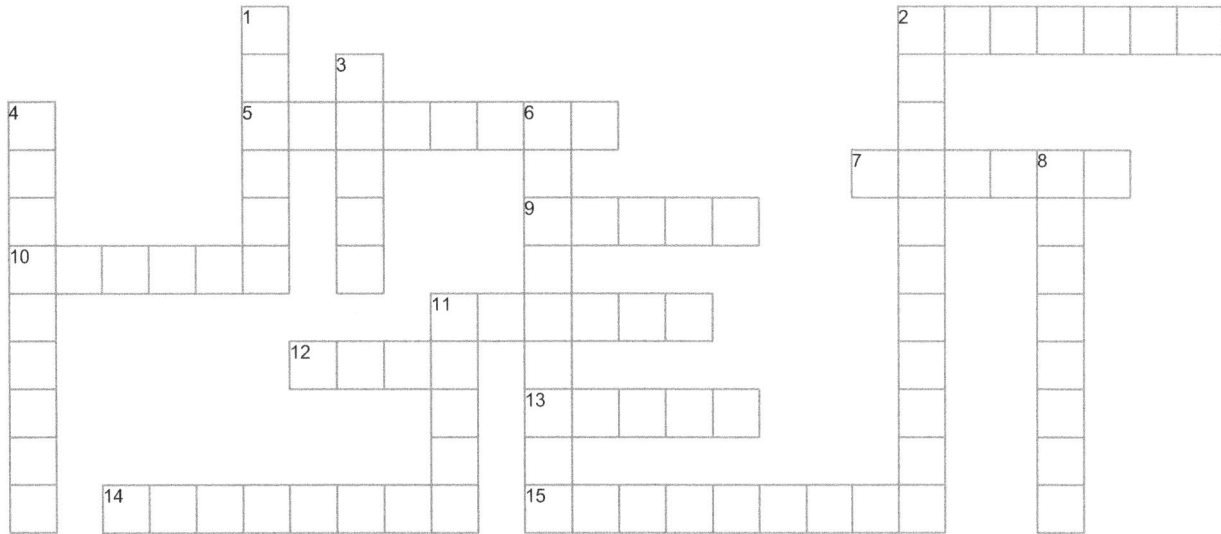

ACROSS

2. Provide exact items; be specific.
5. Tell how things are different; draw a distinction.
7. To make things or ideas known to others; to share or to get ideas across to others.
9. To represent something that will serve as an example.
10. Support; uphold.
11. A group of lines in a poem (similar to a paragraph).
12. To determine and mark points on a graph.
13. to hint at something without saying it.
14. Proof; information in the text that proves a point.
15. Able to do its job to the best ability.

DOWN

1. To put down in writing so that it is saved.
2. Show; make plain.
3. Make a good guess; read between the lines.
4. Helps to support the central idea in an important way. Authors elaborate using examples or anecdotes.
6. Sum it up; give a short version.
8. Stated clearly and in detail.
11. Clearly express something in a speech or writing.

A. Convey	B. Record	C. Summarize	D. Details	E. Defend
F. Evidence	G. Explicit	H. Infer	I. Effective	J. Key detail
K. Demonstrate	L. Stanza	M. Imply	N. Contrast	O. Model
P. State	Q. Plot			

13. *Using the Across and Down clues, write the correct words in the numbered grid below.*

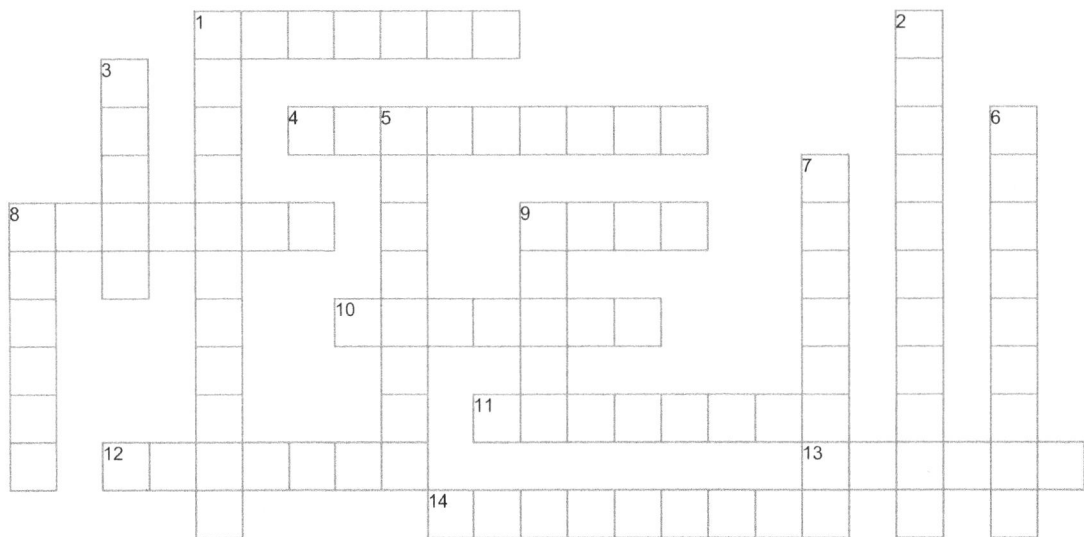

ACROSS

1. A simplified drawing.
4. A story.
8. To think of what will happen in the future or later.
9. Group; classify.
10. Explain how things are the same.
11. A corrected or new version of something written.
12. A usually short piece of written work that focuses on a topic.
13. To make a product.
14. To come up with.

DOWN

1. To tell as different.
2. The main point of the story or the text; the unifying element of a story or text, sometimes called main idea or theme.
3. Name; identify.
5. An answer or reply.
6. Put together; create.
7. Put in order; put in a series.
8. A group of words within a text.
9. Say; affirm.

A. Predict   B. Sequence   C. Formulate   D. Response   E. Distinguish
F. Formulate   G. Revision   H. Phrase   I. Compare   J. Create
K. Diagram   L. Label   M. Central idea N. Passage   O. Narrative
P. Sort   Q. State

14. *Using the Across and Down clues, write the correct words in the numbered grid below.*

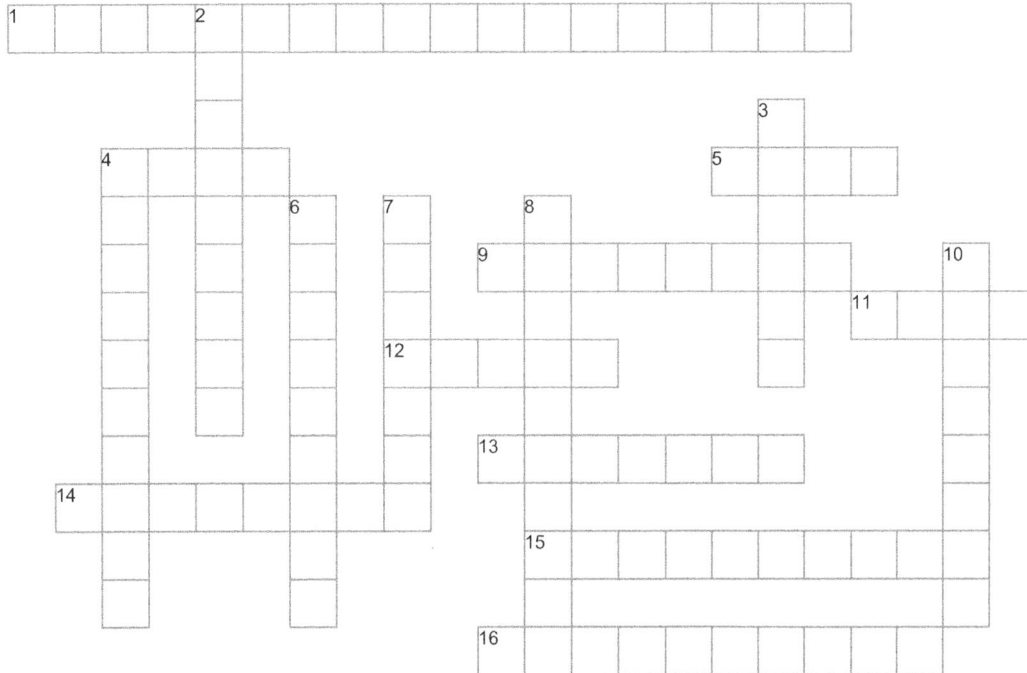

ACROSS

1. Words that may not literally mean what they say.
4. A temporary state of mind or feeling.
5. The reading passage.
9. A person who tells something; storyteller.
11. To determine and mark points on a graph.
12. Name; identify.
13. Tell how alike; judge against.
14. To tell or write about something in detail.
15. To make clear by using examples.
16. The ending, answer, or conclusion to a problem or story.

DOWN

2. To identify from knowledge of appearance or characteristics.
3. To put down in writing so that it is saved.
4. Will probably happen; probably.
6. To show to be true, to prove.
7. Give a rough idea; plan.
8. To put in a group based on certain characteristics.
10. A word, phrase or clause used to describe or qualify another word, phrase or clause.

A. Outline
E. Compare
I. Record
M. Categorize
Q. Narrator

B. Label
F. Modifier
J. Establish
N. Text

C. Figurative language
G. Most likely
K. Recognize
O. Illustrate

D. Mood
H. Resolution
L. Describe
P. Plot

15. *Using the Across and Down clues, write the correct words in the numbered grid below.*

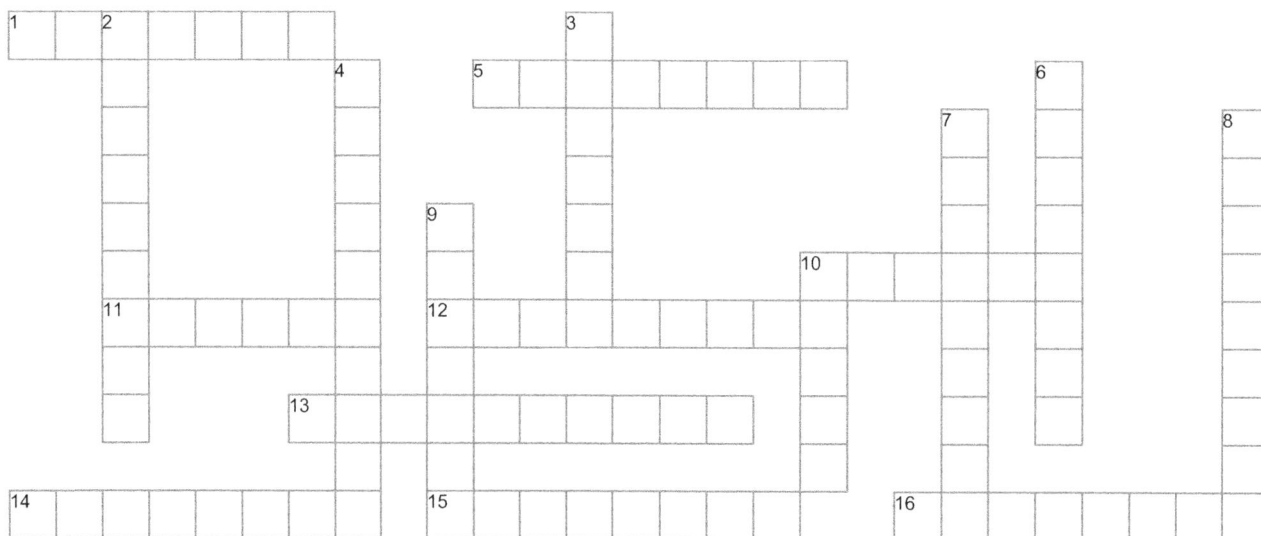

ACROSS

1. To prove.
5. A person who tells something; storyteller.
10. A book, person, or document used to provide information or data.
11. To cause changes.
12. To determine the meaning of.
13. To change something to work in a certain way.
14. To persuade or get someone to think a certain way.
15. Proof; information in the text that proves a point.
16. Tell about; explain.

DOWN

2. Sum it up; give a short version.
3. Exact or specific.
4. To draw or make pictures to explain.
6. Proof; lines and words from text used to prove or disprove an idea.
7. A story.
8. Exaggeration, not meant to be literal.
9. Use something to help find a solution.
10. Say; affirm.

A. Summarize   B. Hyperbole   C. Illustrate   D. Interpret   E. Justify
F. Convince   G. Narrative   H. Utilize   I. Precise   J. Impact
K. Evidence   L. Source   M. Narrator   N. State   O. Evidence
P. Describe   Q. Manipulate

16. *Using the Across and Down clues, write the correct words in the numbered grid below.*

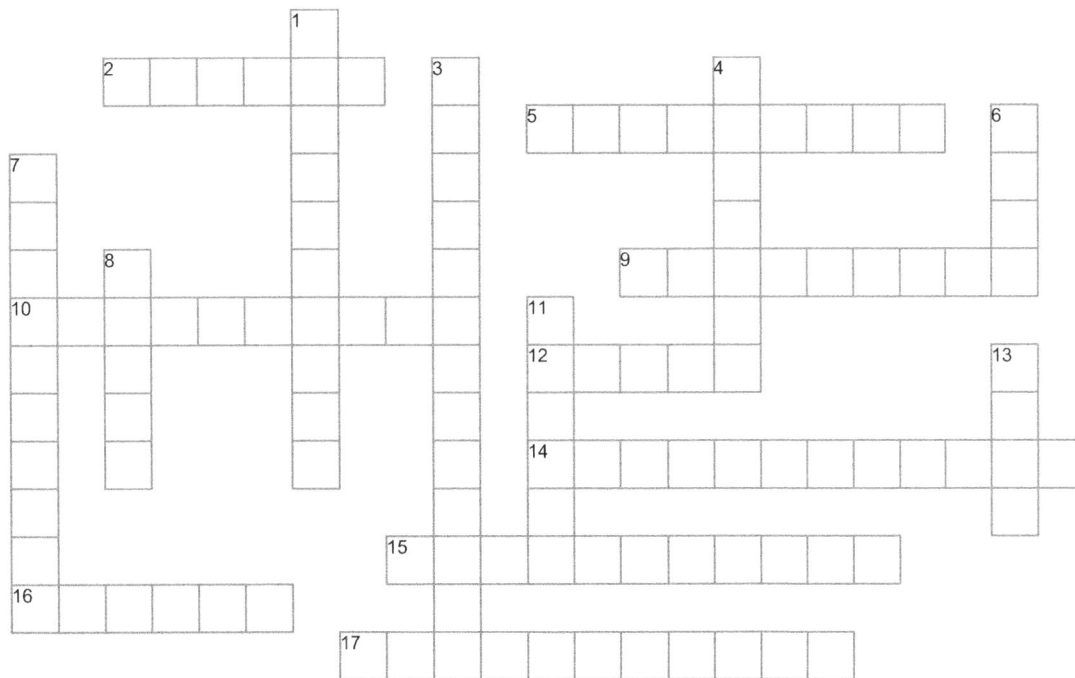

ACROSS

2. The moment in the story where the conflict reaches its highest point.

5. Copy; repeat.

9. A way of looking or thinking about something.

10. To make clear by using examples.

12. Anything that happens, especially something important or unusual.

14. The fact of making something seem larger, more important, better, or worse than it really is; overstate the truth.

15. To tell as different.

16. What happens because of something.

17. All the meanings, associations, emotions, or tones that a word suggests.

DOWN

1. A restatement of the meaning of a text or passage using other words.

3. The meaning a reader gets from written text.

4. To gather together.

6. To determine and mark points on a graph.

7. To change something to work in a certain way.

8. To state a position or declare that something is true or factual, noun-a statement of truth or fact, typically pertaining to an idea that is disputed.

11. To choose.

13. The events that make up the story or the main part of the story. The events relate to each other in a pattern or sequence.

A. Plot
E. Climax
I. Plot
M. Illustrate
Q. Paraphrase

B. Manipulate
F. Distinguish
J. Select
N. Collect

C. Connotation
G. Effect
K. Viewpoint
O. Exaggeration

D. Reproduce
H. Claim
L. Comprehension
P. Event

17. *Using the Across and Down clues, write the correct words in the numbered grid below.*

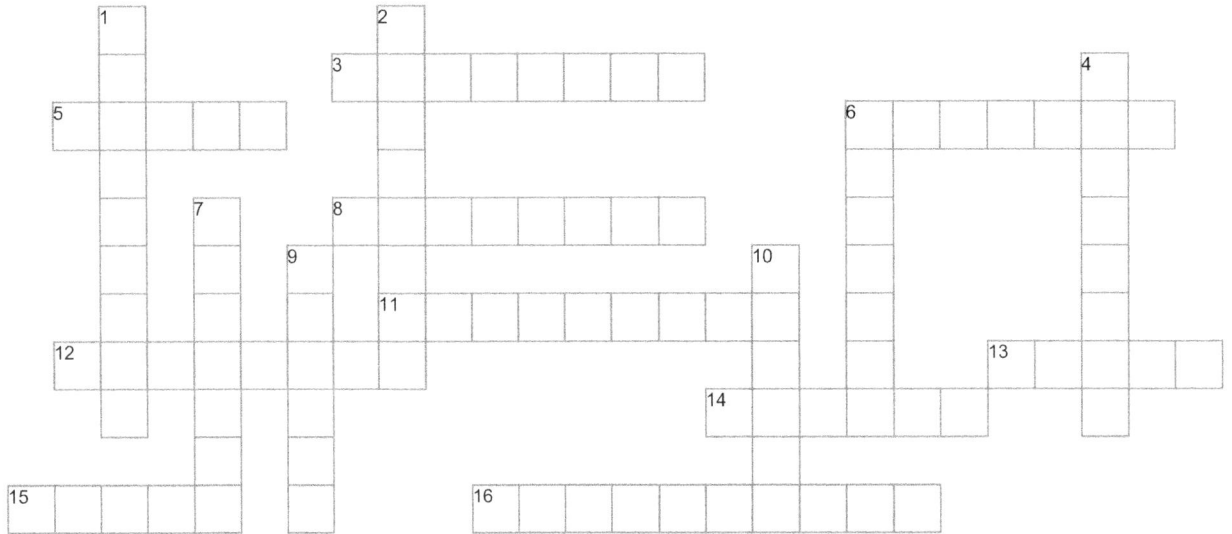

ACROSS

3. To tell or write about something in detail.

5. Plain; rough copy.

6. An explanation for a picture or illustration.

8. A word, phrase or clause used to describe or qualify another word, phrase or clause.

11. Sum it up; give a short version.

12. Judge; consider.

13. A short literary composition on a theme or subject - usually analytic or interpretive in nature.

14. Support; uphold.

15. To produce words.

16. To change something to work in a certain way.

DOWN

1. A story.

2. An answer or reply.

4. To find differences.

6. Explain how things are the same.

7. Use something to help find a solution.

9. A group of lines forming the basic unit in a poem; a verse.

10. To show or make known.

A. Modifier   B. Evaluate   C. Describe   D. Compare   E. Contrast
F. Essay   G. Manipulate   H. Caption   I. Response   J. Write
K. Stanza   L. Narrative   M. Reveal   N. Summarize   O. Draft
P. Utilize   Q. Defend

18. *Using the Across and Down clues, write the correct words in the numbered grid below.*

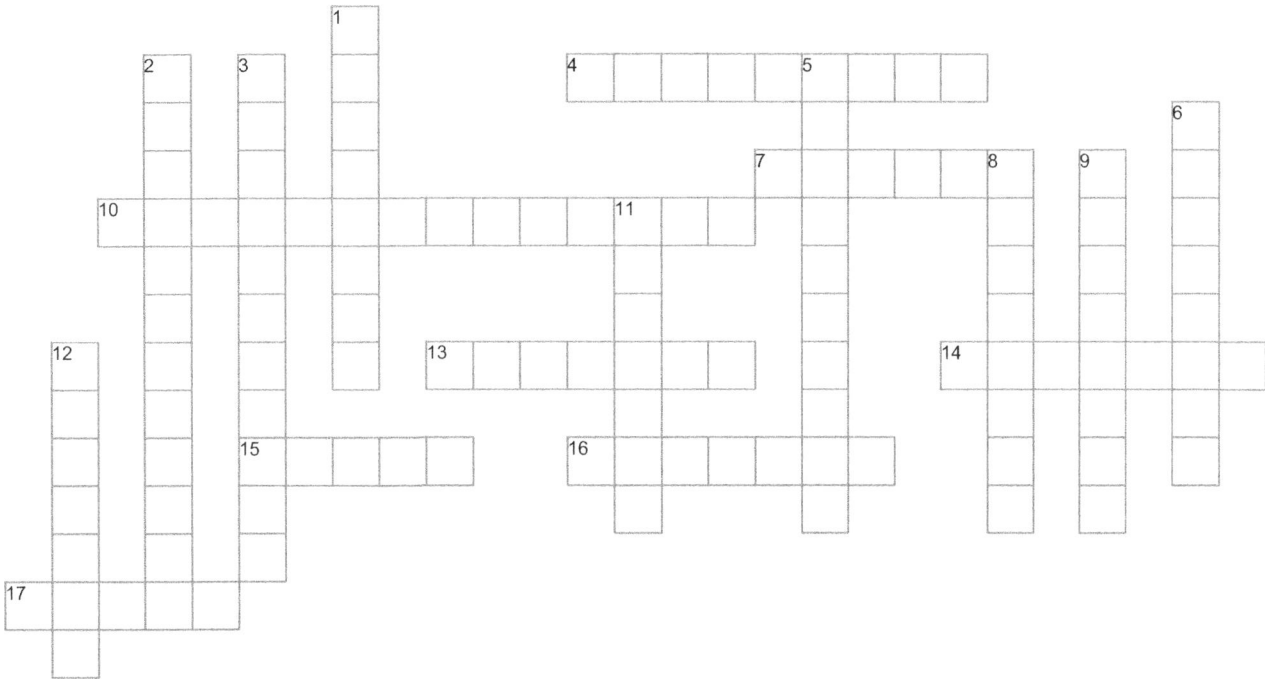

ACROSS

4. Explain the meaning; make clear.
7. To make a product.
10. Read and examine text in detail looking for important ideas.
13. Not true.
14. Repeat; say again.
15. Make a good guess; read between the lines.
16. Talk about; argue.
17. Sort; organize.

DOWN

1. A corrected or new version of something written.
2. A part of the story that is important.
3. Data that is based on numbers.
5. A restatement of the meaning of a text or passage using other words.
6. A person who tells something; storyteller.
8. Proof; information in the text that proves a point.
9. Job, what it does.
11. Make clear; put in your own words.
12. To provide proof or evidence for.

A. Significance   B. Invalid   C. Paraphrase   D. Explain
E. Analysis of text F. Function   G. Revision   H. Evidence
I. Narrator   J. Support   K. Order   L. Interpret
M. Discuss   N. Create   O. Qualitative   P. Restate
Q. Infer

19. *Using the Across and Down clues, write the correct words in the numbered grid below.*

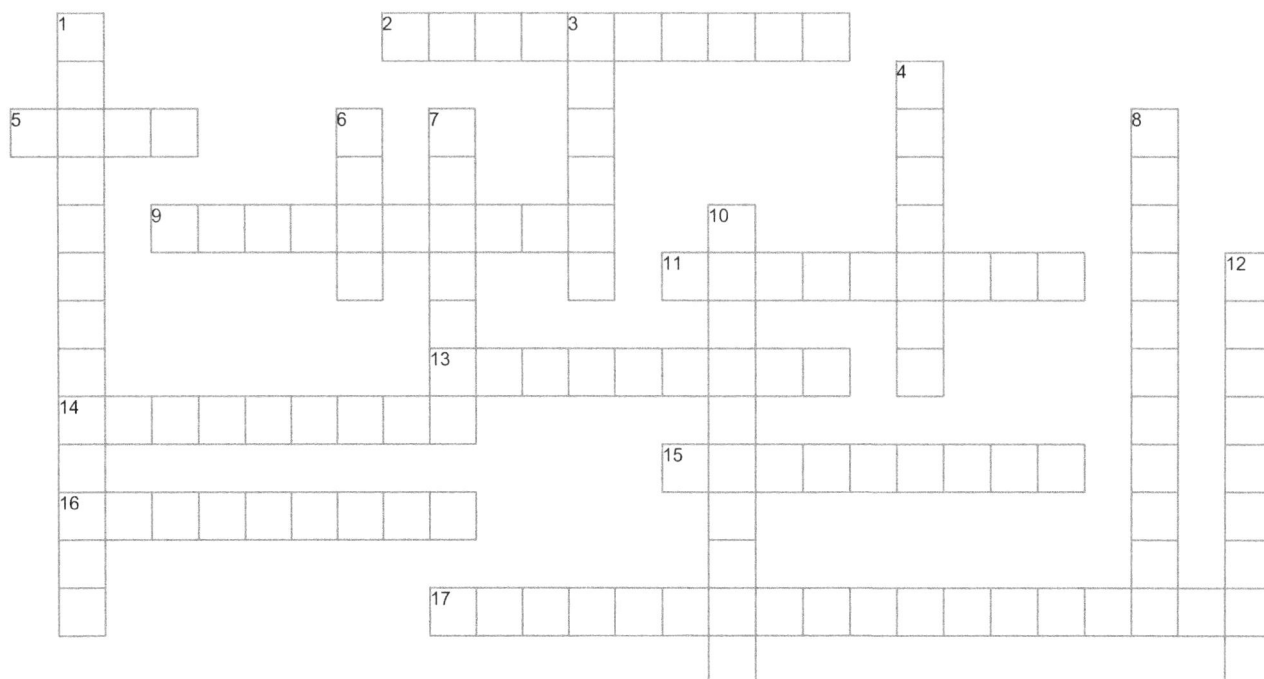

ACROSS

2. to make a statement based upon details from the reading passage that might be true in other situations.

5. A temporary state of mind or feeling.

9. To draw or make pictures to explain.

11. A section of writing consisting of one or more sentences grouped together and discussing one main subject.

13. To paraphrase or to explain in your own words an important idea or section of text.

14. A story.

15. Sum it up; give a short version.

16. To relate to concepts.

17. Words or expression different from literal language, changed or altered to make a linguistic point.

DOWN

1. A punctuation mark ", " or ',' used at the beginning and ending of text that has been stated from a source.

3. Look at; study.

4. Watch; notice.

6. Record; name.

7. The reason someone does something.

8. The main point of the story or the text; the unifying element of a story or text, sometimes called main idea or theme.

10. To change something to work in a certain way.

12. To think about carefully and form an opinion.

A. Narrative   B. List   C. Generalize   D. Central idea
E. Paragraph   F. Manipulate   G. Observe   H. Associate
I. Purpose   J. Summarize   K. Summarize   L. Mood
M. Concludes   N. Illustrate   O. Review   P. Figurative language
Q. Quotation mark

20. *Using the Across and Down clues, write the correct words in the numbered grid below.*

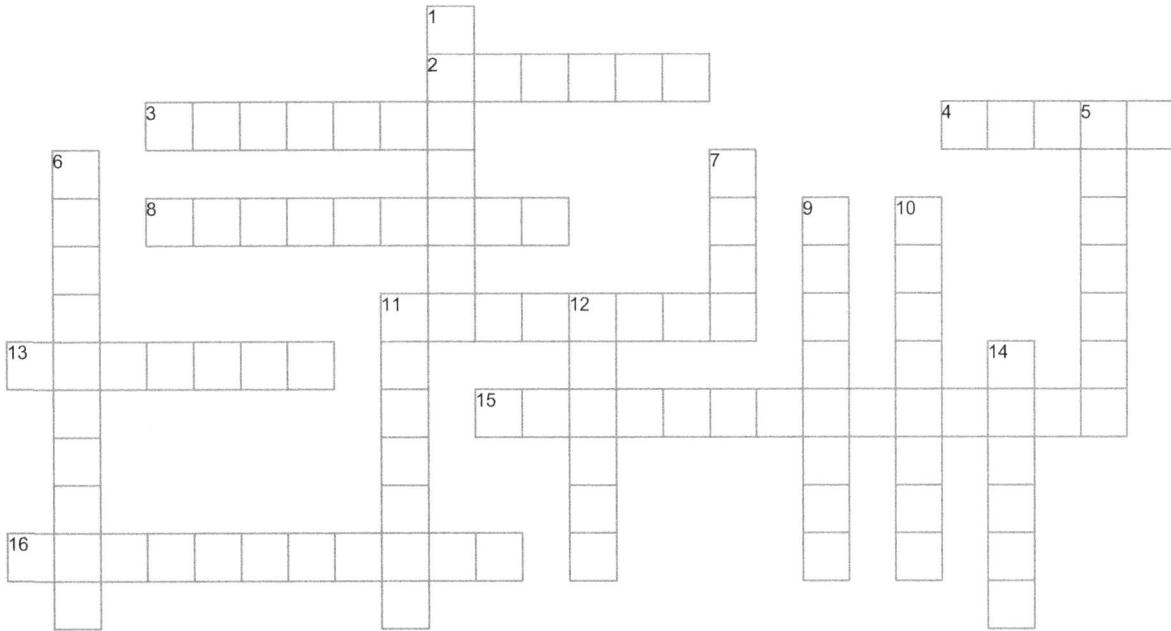

ACROSS

2. Change; alter.
3. The reason someone does something.
4. A short literary composition on a theme or subject - usually analytic or interpretive in nature.
8. Sum it up; give a short version.
11. Tell about; explain.
13. To consider an idea.
15. Reason the author writes: persuade, inform, entertain (PIE).
16. To search for an answer to a solution.

DOWN

1. Exact or specific.
5. Break apart; study the pieces.
6. To do something the same constantly.
7. To use a quote from the text to support an idea.
9. A comparison of two unlike things by describing one is the other.
10. To tell or write about something in detail.
11. A simplified drawing.
12. Repeat; say again.
14. To make things or ideas known to others; to share or to get ideas across to others.

A. Metaphor
B. Precise
C. Convey
D. Revise
E. Authors purpose
F. Discuss
G. Summarize
H. Analyze
I. Diagram
J. Describe
K. Retell
L. Describe
M. Investigate
N. Purpose
O. Essay
P. Consistent
Q. Cite

1. *Using the Across and Down clues, write the correct words in the numbered grid below.*

ACROSS

3. Judge; consider.
7. Guess; tell what will happen next.
9. Use details from the text to explain your response.
10. A simplified drawing.
11. To come up with.
13. To produce words.
14. To draw or make pictures to explain.
15. A sentence that pulls together or summarizes the main idea and provides a definite ending point for a paragraph or written piece.
16. Make out; break apart.

DOWN

1. Text that the author presents as an argument.
2. The way a text is presented: introduction, headings and
4. A comparison of two unlike things by describing one is the other.
5. To make a product.
6. The way someone feels about something.
8. A word, phrase or clause used to describe or qualify another word, phrase or clause.
10. A single piece of information or fact about something.
12. Break apart; study the pieces.

A. Textual evidence   B. Attitude
E. Predict   F. Evaluate
I. Support   J. Detail
M. Text structure   N. Construct
Q. Formulate

C. Modifier   D. Analyze
G. Illustrate   H. Write
K. Decode   L. Diagram
O. Concluding sentence   P. Metaphor

2. *Using the Across and Down clues, write the correct words in the numbered grid below.*

¹S	E	Q	U	E	N	C	E											²R	
U																		E	
³M	O	S	T	L	I	K	E	⁴L	Y		⁵C	O	N	C	⁶L	U	D	E	S
M							A						E		⁷I			P		R
A							B						N		N			R		O
R			⁸C				E				⁹R		O		F			D		U
Y		¹⁰C	O	N	C	L	¹¹U	D	I	N	G	S	E	N	T	E	N	C	E
			N				T				E			T	A			R		U
¹²N	A	R	R	A	T	O	R				E			T	I		¹³P	R	E	C	I	S	E
			R				I				L			L	I			N	
	¹⁴S	U	M	M	A	R	Y				L			L	O			C	
			S				Z								N			E	
¹⁵E	V	E	N	T		¹⁶E	V	A	L	U	A	T	E						

ACROSS

1. Order in which events, movements, or things follow each other.
3. Will probably happen; probably.
5. To think about carefully and form an opinion.
10. A sentence that pulls together or summarizes the main idea and provides a definite ending point for a paragraph or written piece.
12. A person who tells something; storyteller.
13. Exact or specific.
14. Using few words to give the most important information about something or a complete but brief account of things previously stated.
15. Anything that happens, especially something important or unusual.
16. Judge; consider.

DOWN

1. A short way of saying what the reading passage is about.
2. Copy; repeat.
4. Name; identify.
6. The basic definition or dictionary meaning of a word.
7. A conclusion reached based on reasoning and the use of given facts; a prediction.
8. To find differences.
9. Repeat; say again.
11. Use something to help find a solution.

A. Summary
E. Most likely
I. Denotation
M. Sequence
Q. Inference

B. Contrast
F. Retell
J. Precise
N. Utilize

C. Evaluate
G. Concludes
K. Reproduce
O. Narrator

D. Label
H. Summary
L. Event
P. Concluding sentence

3. *Using the Across and Down clues, write the correct words in the numbered grid below.*

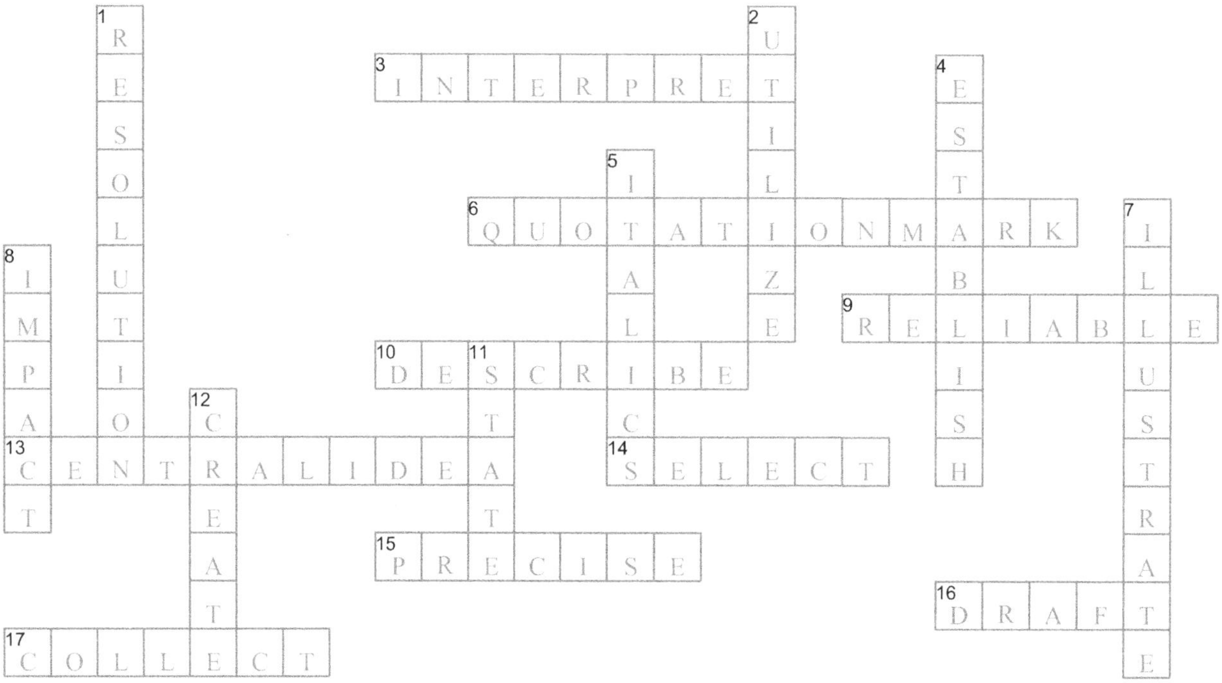
1 RESOLUTION
2 UTILIZE
3 INTERPRET
4 ESTABLISH
5 ITALICS
6 QUOTATIONMARK
7 ILLUSTRATE
8 IMPACT
9 RELIABLE
10 DESCRIBE
11 STATE
12 CREATE
13 CENTRALIDEA
14 SELECT
15 PRECISE
16 DRAFT
17 COLLECT

ACROSS

3. To determine the meaning of.
6. A punctuation mark ", " or ',' used at the beginning and ending of text that has been stated from a source.
9. Able to trust.
10. To tell or write about something in detail.
13. The main point of the story or the text; the unifying element of a story or text, sometimes called main idea or theme.
14. To choose.
15. Exact or specific.
16. Plain; rough copy.
17. To gather together.

DOWN

1. The ending, answer, or conclusion to a problem or story.
2. Use something to help find a solution.
4. To show to be true, to prove.
5. A style of print where the letters slope to the right; may be used to emphasize or to indicate the title of published work.
7. To draw or make pictures to explain.
8. To cause changes.
11. Say; affirm.
12. To make a product.

A. Illustrate	B. Precise	C. Utilize	D. State
E. Resolution	F. Reliable	G. Collect	H. Select
I. Describe	J. Italics	K. Draft	L. Central idea
M. Impact	N. Establish	O. Interpret	P. Create
Q. Quotation mark			

4. *Using the Across and Down clues, write the correct words in the numbered grid below.*

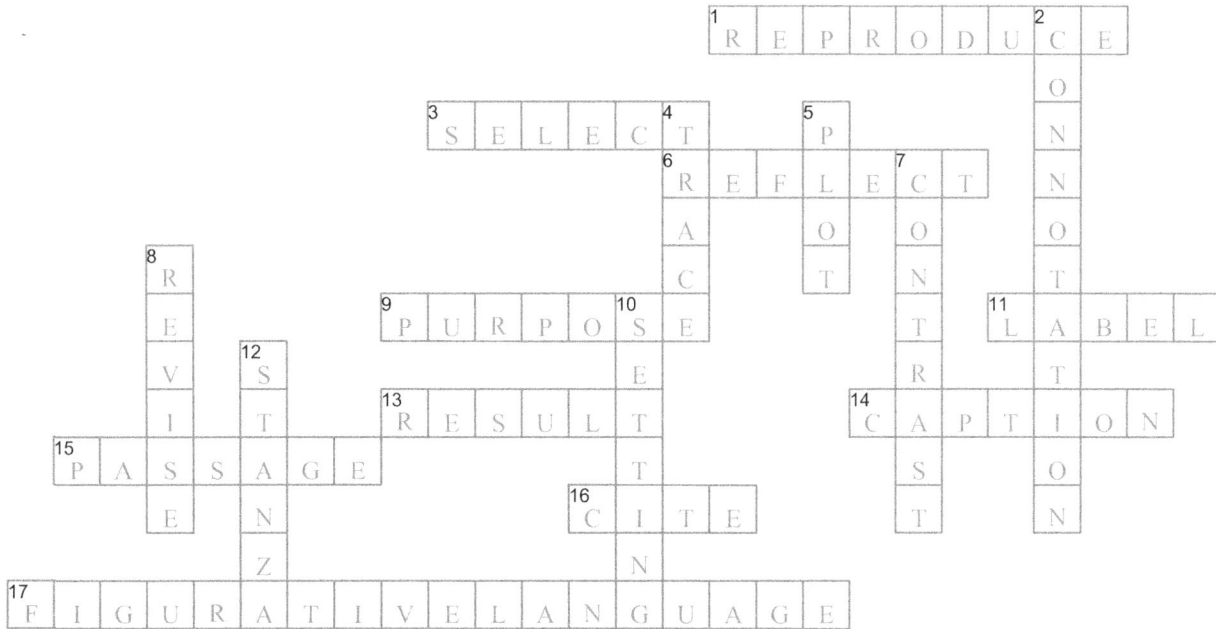

```
                                              1                           2
                                              R  E  P  R  O  D  U  C  E
                                                                       O
              3           4          5                                 N
              S  E  L  E  C  T        P                                N
                                 6                    7
                                 R  E  F  L  E  C  T                   O
                                 A        O     O                      T
                                 C        T     N           11
       8                   9              10                L  A  B  E  L
       R                   P  U  R  P  O  S  E              T
       E         12                      E                 R
       V         S            13                 14        T
       I         T            R  E  S  U  L  T    C  A  P  T  I  O  N
   15                                     T       A        S
       P  A  S  S  A  G  E         16             P        O
       E         N            C  I  T  E          T        N
                 Z                        N       T
   17
       F  I  G  U  R  A  T  I  V  E  L  A  N  G  U  A  G  E
```

ACROSS

1. Copy; repeat.
3. To choose.
6. Think about; wonder about.
9. The reason someone does something.
11. Name; identify.
13. Give an answer; consequence.
14. An explanation for a picture or illustration.
15. Part; section.
16. To use a quote from the text to support an idea.
17. Words or expression different from literal language, changed or altered to make a linguistic point.

DOWN

2. All the meanings, associations, emotions, or tones that a word suggests.
4. Outline; map out.
5. The events that make up the story or the main part of the story. The events relate to each other in a pattern or sequence.
7. To find differences.
8. Change; alter.
10. The period and-or location in which a story takes place.
12. A group of lines in a poem (similar to a paragraph).

A. Result
B. Contrast
C. Stanza
D. Setting
E. Select
F. Reproduce
G. Reflect
H. Revise
I. Connotation
J. Passage
K. Plot
L. Cite
M. Trace
N. Label
O. Figurative language
P. Purpose
Q. Caption

5. *Using the Across and Down clues, write the correct words in the numbered grid below.*

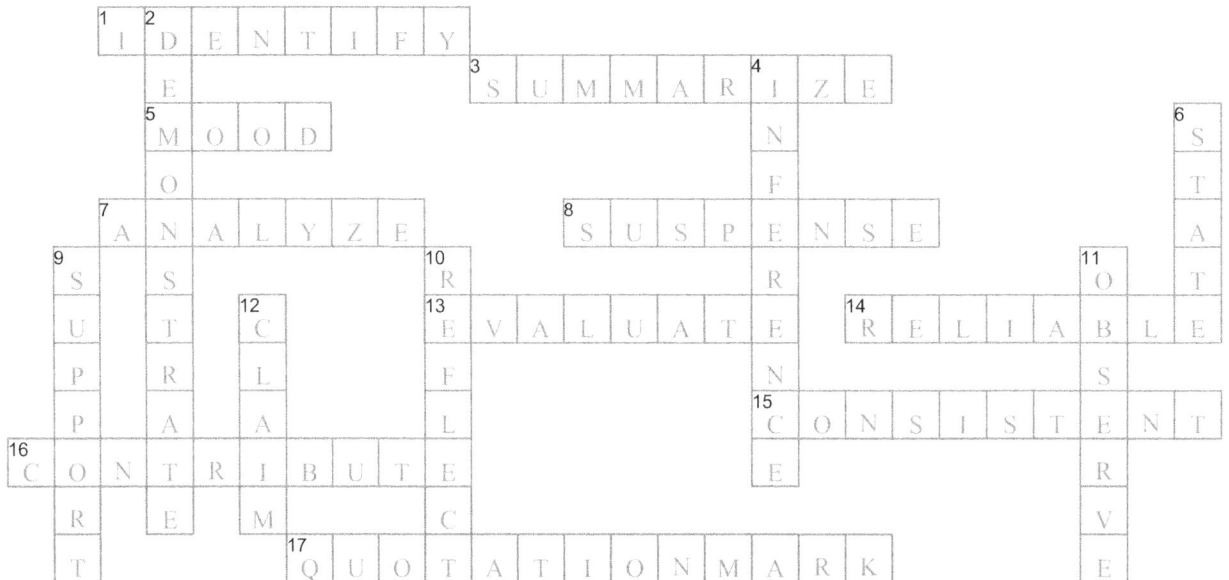

¹I	²D	E	N	T	I	F	Y					
	E					³S	U	M	M	A	R	⁴I	Z	E

(Crossword grid)

I D E N T I F Y
³S U M M A R I Z E
⁵M O O D
⁷A N A L Y Z E ⁸S U S P E N S E
¹³E V A L U A T E ¹⁴R E L I A B L E
¹⁵C O N S I S T E N T
¹⁶C O N T R I B U T E
¹⁷Q U O T A T I O N M A R K

Down words:
2 DEMONSTRATE
4 INFERENCE
6 STATE
9 SUPPORT
10 REFLECT
11 OBSERVE
12 CLAIM

ACROSS

1. Name; label.
3. Sum it up; give a short version.
5. A temporary state of mind or feeling.
7. Break apart; study the pieces.
8. Not sure what is going to happen, waiting.
13. To judge or determine the quality or amount of something.
14. Able to trust.
15. To do something the same constantly.
16. To help happen or help cause.
17. A punctuation mark " , " or ',' used at the beginning and ending of text that has been stated from a source.

DOWN

2. Show; make plain.
4. To come up with a conclusion without valid evidence to support it.
6. Say; affirm.
9. To provide proof or evidence for.
10. Think about; wonder about.
11. Watch; notice.
12. To state a position or declare that something is true or factual, noun-a statement of truth or fact, typically pertaining to an idea that is disputed.

A. Reliable   B. Consistent   C. Inference   D. Identify
E. Mood   F. State   G. Quotation mark   H. Support
I. Evaluate   J. Reflect   K. Observe   L. Analyze
M. Contribute   N. Suspense   O. Summarize   P. Claim
Q. Demonstrate

6. *Using the Across and Down clues, write the correct words in the numbered grid below.*

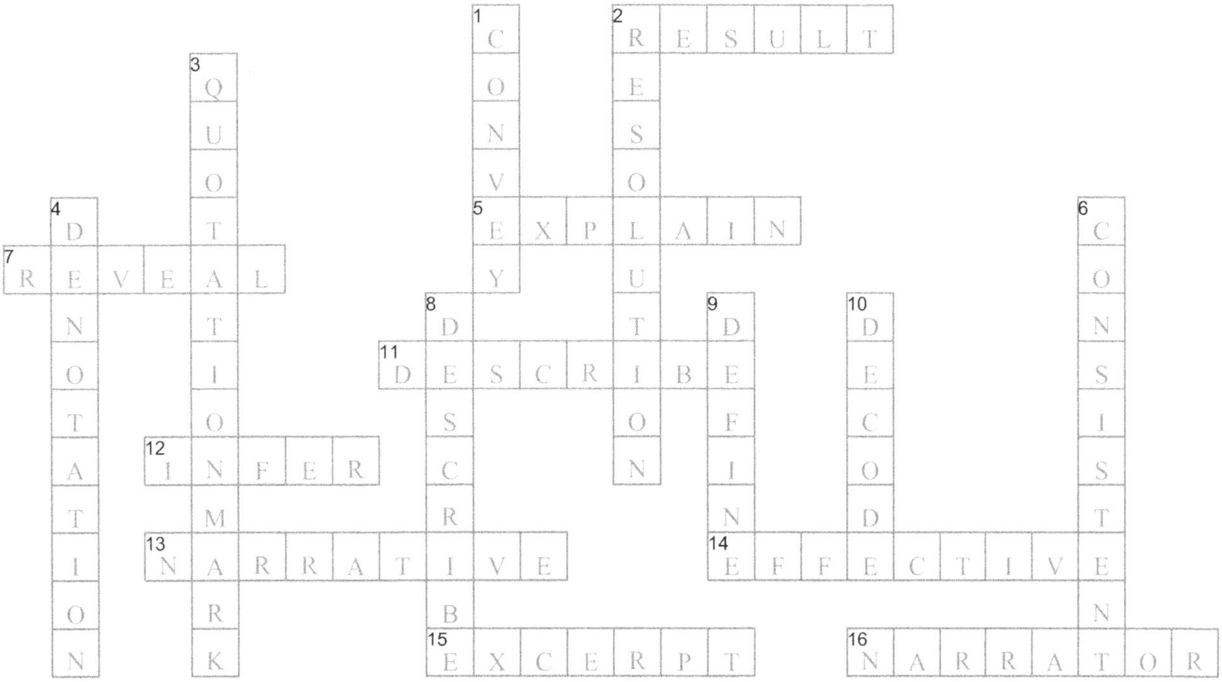
1 CONVEY
2 RESULT
2 RESOLUTION
3 QUOTATION MARK
4 DENOTATION
5 EXPLAIN
6 CONSISTENT
7 REVEAL
8 DESCRIBE
9 DEFINE
10 DECODE
11 DESCRIBE
12 INFER
13 NARRATIVE
14 EFFECTIVE
15 EXCERPT
16 NARRATOR

ACROSS

2. Give an answer; consequence.
5. To give details to make something clear.
7. To show or make known.
11. Tell about; explain.
12. To explain an idea or make a conclusion by looking closely at evidence in text.
13. A story.
14. Able to do its job to the best ability.
15. A part of a reading passage.
16. A person who tells something; storyteller.

DOWN

1. To make things or ideas known to others; to share or to get ideas across to others.
2. The ending, answer, or conclusion to a problem or story.
3. A punctuation mark ", " or ',' used at the beginning and ending of text that has been stated from a source.
4. The basic definition or dictionary meaning of a word.
6. To do something the same constantly.
8. To tell or write about something in detail.
9. Describe; characterize.
10. Make out; break apart.

A. Decode
B. Narrator
C. Result
D. Resolution
E. Define
F. Consistent
G. Excerpt
H. Describe
I. Infer
J. Reveal
K. Denotation
L. Explain
M. Quotation mark
N. Convey
O. Narrative
P. Describe
Q. Effective

7. *Using the Across and Down clues, write the correct words in the numbered grid below.*

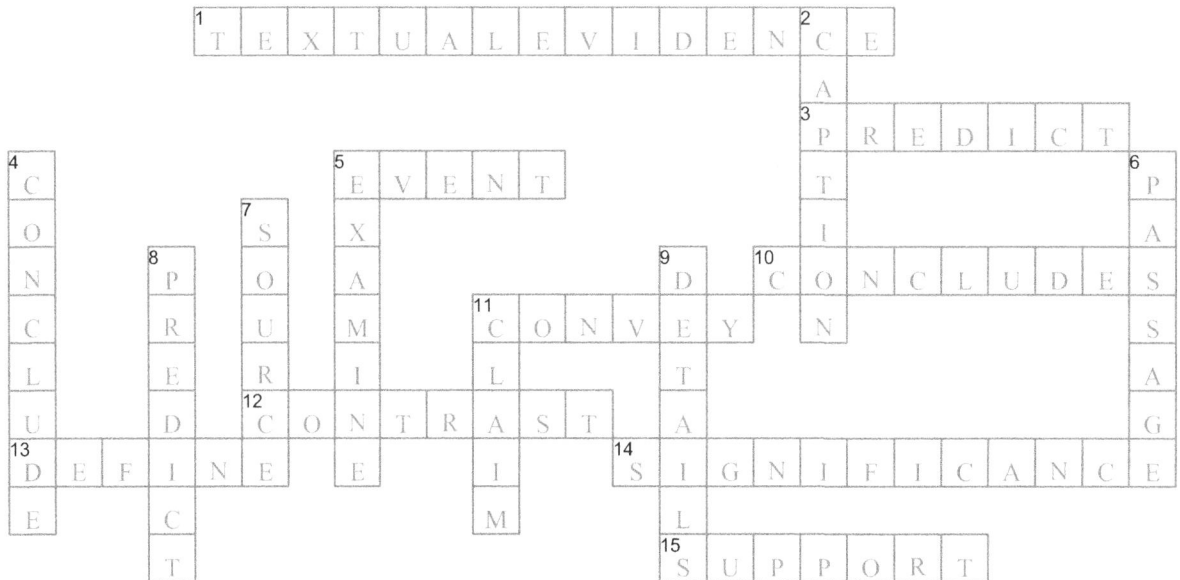

Crossword grid solution:
- 1 Across: TEXTUAL EVIDENCE
- 2 Down: CAPTION
- 3 Across: PREDICT
- 4 Down: CONCLUDE
- 5 Across: EVENT
- 5 Down: EXAMINE
- 6 Down: PASSAGE
- 7 Down: SOURCE
- 8 Down: PREDICT
- 9 Down: DEFINE
- 10 Across: CONCLUDES
- 11 Across: CONVEY
- 11 Down: CLAIM
- 12 Across: CONTRAST
- 13 Across: DEFINE
- 14 Across: SIGNIFICANCE
- 15 Across: SUPPORT

ACROSS

1. Text that the author presents as an argument.
3. To think of what will happen in the future or later.
5. Anything that happens, especially something important or unusual.
10. To think about carefully and form an opinion.
11. To make things or ideas known to others; to share or to get ideas across to others.
12. Explain how things are different.
13. Describe; characterize.
14. A part of the story that is important.
15. Give the facts; back up with details.

DOWN

2. An explanation for a picture or illustration.
4. to decide based upon information stated in the reading passages.
5. Look at; inspect.
6. A usually short piece of written work that focuses on a topic.
7. A book, person, or document used to provide information or data.
8. Guess; tell what will happen next.
9. Provide exact items; be specific.
11. To state a position or declare that something is true or factual, noun-a statement of truth or fact, typically pertaining to an idea that is disputed.

A. Event
E. Details
I. Predict
M. Concludes
Q. Passage

B. Source
F. Contrast
J. Support
N. Examine

C. Significance
G. Textual evidence
K. Conclude
O. Predict

D. Claim
H. Convey
L. Caption
P. Define

8. *Using the Across and Down clues, write the correct words in the numbered grid below.*

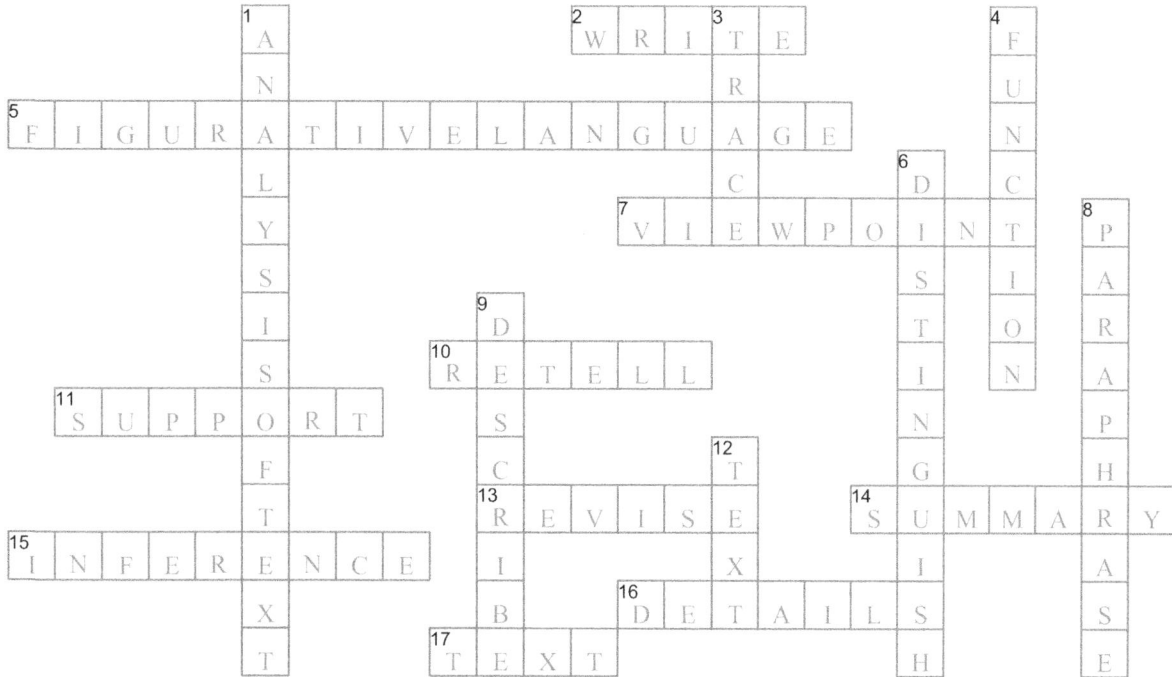

The crossword grid contains the following filled answers:

- 2 Across: WRITE
- 5 Across: FIGURATIVELANGUAGE
- 7 Across: VIEWPOINT
- 10 Across: RETELL
- 11 Across: SUPPORT
- 13 Across: REVISE
- 14 Across: SUMMARY
- 15 Across: INFERENCE
- 16 Across: DETAILS
- 17 Across: TEXT
- 1 Down: ANALYSIST (ANALYSISOFTEXT)
- 3 Down: TRCD (TRACED...)
- 4 Down: FUNCTION
- 6 Down: DISTINGUISH
- 8 Down: PARAPHRASE
- 9 Down: DESCRIB
- 12 Down: TEXT

ACROSS

2. To produce words.
5. Words that may not literally mean what they say.
7. A way of looking or thinking about something.
10. Repeat; say again.
11. Use details from the text to explain your response.
13. Change; alter.
14. A short way of saying what the reading passage is about.
15. To come up with a conclusion without valid evidence to support it.
16. Provide exact items; be specific.
17. A book or other written work or printed work.

DOWN

1. Read and examine text in detail looking for important ideas.
3. Outline; map out.
4. Job, what it does.
6. To tell as different.
8. A restatement of the meaning of a text or passage using other words.
9. Tell about; explain.
12. The reading passage.

A. Trace
E. Distinguish
I. Analysis of text
M. Write
Q. Viewpoint

B. Revise
F. Support
J. Summary
N. Figurative language

C. Text
G. Text
K. Details
O. Paraphrase

D. Retell
H. Function
L. Describe
P. Inference

9. *Using the Across and Down clues, write the correct words in the numbered grid below.*

		¹I	²N	T	E	R	P	R	E	T		³A	⁴S	S	⁵E	S	S
⁶K			O				A						U		U		
E			⁸R	E	C	O	R	D					S		P		
Y			G				R		⁹T				P		P		
D			A			¹⁰V	I	¹¹S	U	A	L	I	Z	E	O		
E			N				¹²T	E	X	T			N		R		
T			I					¹³C	O	L	L	¹⁴E	C	T	S		
¹⁵A	N	A	L	Y	Z	E		V			E		I		E		
I			E			¹⁶E	V	I	D	E	N	C	E				
¹⁷L	A	B	E	L				T				E					

ACROSS

1. Explain the meaning; make clear.
3. Judge; consider.
8. To put down in writing so that it is saved.
10. Imagine; think about.
12. A book or other written work or printed work.
13. To gather together.
15. To look at text carefully by paying attention to its parts, its words, its figurative language, and its tone.
16. Proof; information in the text that proves a point.
17. Name; identify.

DOWN

2. A story.
4. Not sure what is going to happen, waiting.
5. Give the facts; back up with details.
6. Helps to support the central idea in an important way. Authors elaborate using examples or anecdotes.
7. Put in order; arrange.
9. The reading passage.
11. To choose.
14. To use a quote from the text to support an idea.

A. Suspense   B. Record   C. Analyze   D. Visualize   E. Interpret   F. Text
G. Collect   H. Assess   I. Organize   J. Label   K. Evidence   L. Text
M. Select   N. Key detail O. Narrative P. Cite   Q. Support

10. *Using the Across and Down clues, write the correct words in the numbered grid below.*

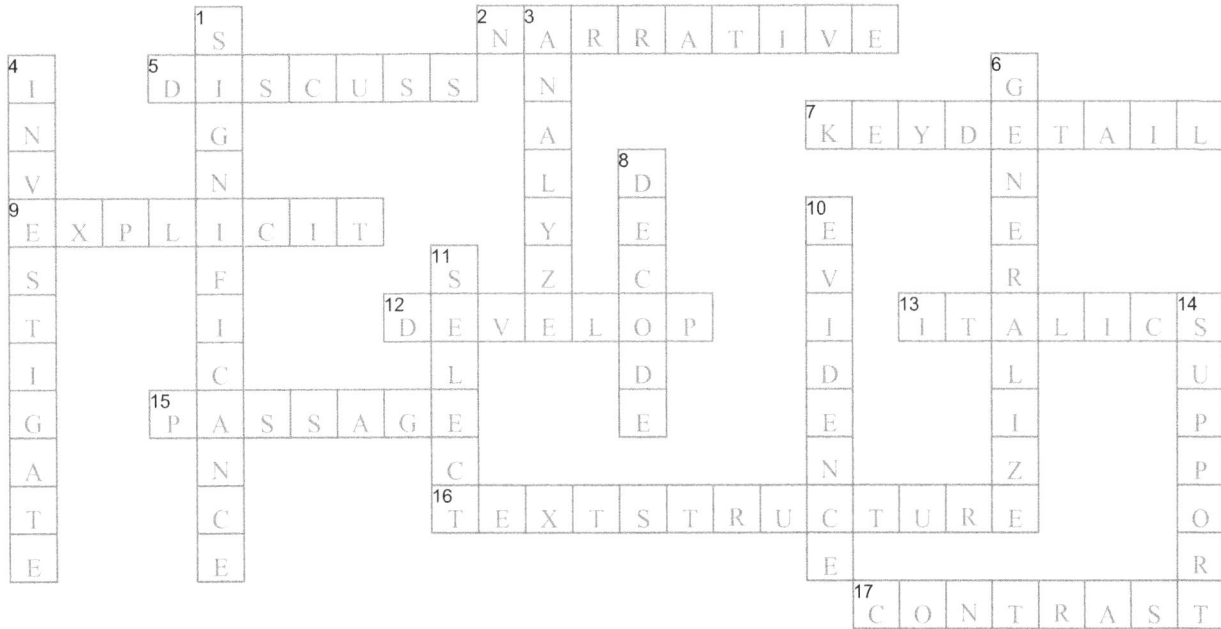

Grid answers:

- 1 Down: INVESTIGATE
- 2 Across: NARRATIVE
- 3 Down: ANALYZE
- 4 Down: INVESTIGATE
- 5 Across/Down: DISCUSS / SIGNIFICANCE
- 6 Down: GENERALIZE
- 7 Across: KEY DETAIL
- 8 Down: DECODE
- 9 Across: EXPLICIT
- 10 Down: EVIDENCE
- 11 Down: SELECT
- 12 Across: DEVELOP
- 13 Across: ITALICS
- 14 Down: SUPPORT
- 15 Across: PASSAGE
- 16 Across: TEXT STRUCTURE
- 17 Across: CONTRAST

ACROSS

2. A story.

5. To consider an idea.

7. Helps to support the central idea in an important way. Authors elaborate using examples or anecdotes.

9. Stated clearly and in detail.

12. To work out, grow, or expand.

13. A style of print where the letters slope to the right; may be used to emphasize or to indicate the title of published work.

15. Part; section.

16. The way a text is presented: introduction, headings and

17. Explain how things are different.

DOWN

1. A part of the story that is important.

3. Break apart; study the pieces.

4. To search for an answer to a solution.

6. to make a statement based upon details from the reading passage that might be true in other situations.

8. Make out; break apart.

10. Proof; information in the text that proves a point.

11. To choose.

14. Give the facts; back up with details.

A. Explicit
F. Contrast
K. Analyze
P. Support

B. Evidence
G. Italics
L. Text structure
Q. Investigate

C. Significance
H. Discuss
M. Develop

D. Key detail
I. Select
N. Decode

E. Generalize
J. Narrative
O. Passage

11. *Using the Across and Down clues, write the correct words in the numbered grid below.*

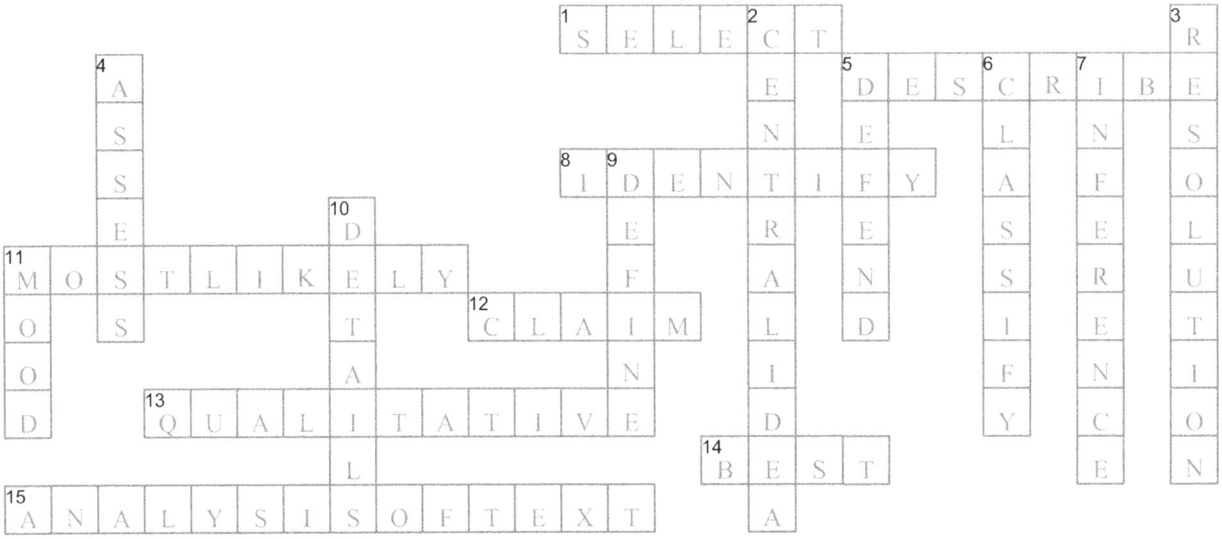

Crossword grid answers:
- 1 Across: SELECT
- 5 Across: DESCRIBE
- 8 Across: IDENTIFY
- 11 Across: MOSTLIKELY
- 12 Across: CLAIM
- 13 Across: QUALITATIVE
- 14 Across: BEST
- 15 Across: ANALYSISOFTEXT
- 2 Down: CENTRALIDEA
- 3 Down: RESOLUTION
- 4 Down: ASSESS
- 5 Down: DEFEND
- 6 Down: CLASSIFY
- 7 Down: INFERENCE
- 9 Down: DESCRIBE
- 10 Down: DETAIL
- 11 Down: MOOD

ACROSS

1. To choose.

5. To tell the facts, details.

8. To recognize or establish as being a person or thing.

11. Will probably happen; probably.

12. To state a position or declare that something is true or factual, noun-a statement of truth or fact, typically pertaining to an idea that is disputed.

13. Data that is based on numbers.

14. Above all others, most desirable.

15. Read and examine text in detail looking for important ideas.

DOWN

2. The main point of the story or the text; the unifying element of a story or text, sometimes called main idea or theme.

3. The ending, answer, or conclusion to a problem or story.

4. Judge; consider.

5. Support; uphold.

6. Put in order; sort.

7. To come up with a conclusion without valid evidence to support it.

9. Describe; characterize.

10. Provide exact items; be specific.

11. A temporary state of mind or feeling.

A. Details
E. Claim
I. Most likely
M. Classify
Q. Defend

B. Resolution
F. Mood
J. Select
N. Best

C. Analysis of text
G. Define
K. Inference
O. Identify

D. Central idea
H. Assess
L. Qualitative
P. Describe

12. *Using the Across and Down clues, write the correct words in the numbered grid below.*

ACROSS

2. Provide exact items; be specific.
5. Tell how things are different; draw a distinction.
7. To make things or ideas known to others; to share or to get ideas across to others.
9. To represent something that will serve as an example.
10. Support; uphold.
11. A group of lines in a poem (similar to a paragraph).
12. To determine and mark points on a graph.
13. to hint at something without saying it.
14. Proof; information in the text that proves a point.
15. Able to do its job to the best ability.

DOWN

1. To put down in writing so that it is saved.
2. Show; make plain.
3. Make a good guess; read between the lines.
4. Helps to support the central idea in an important way. Authors elaborate using examples or anecdotes.
6. Sum it up; give a short version.
8. Stated clearly and in detail.
11. Clearly express something in a speech or writing.

A. Convey	B. Record	C. Summarize	D. Details	E. Defend
F. Evidence	G. Explicit	H. Infer	I. Effective	J. Key detail
K. Demonstrate	L. Stanza	M. Imply	N. Contrast	O. Model
P. State	Q. Plot			

13. *Using the Across and Down clues, write the correct words in the numbered grid below.*

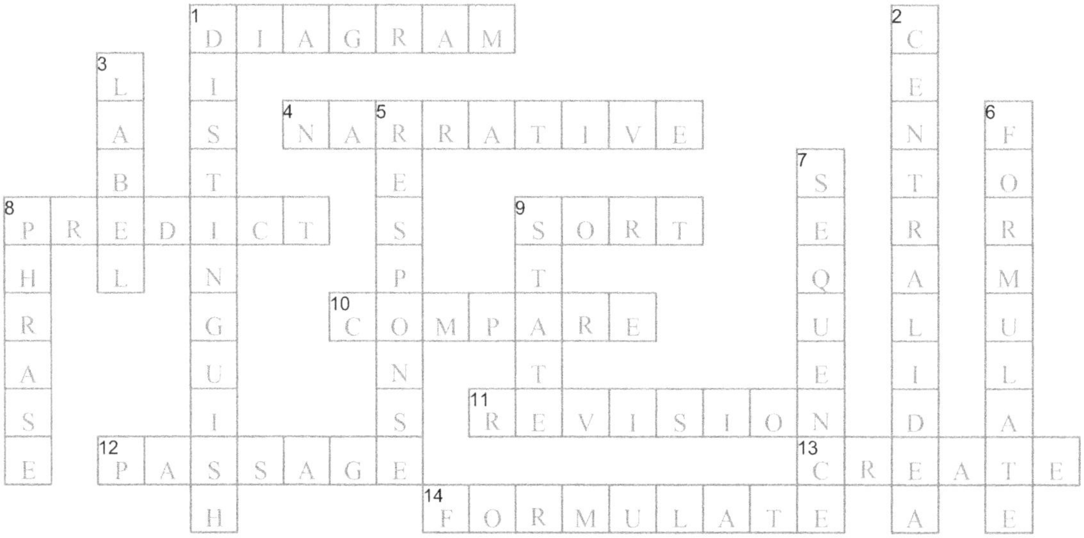

ACROSS

1. A simplified drawing.
4. A story.
8. To think of what will happen in the future or later.
9. Group; classify.
10. Explain how things are the same.
11. A corrected or new version of something written.
12. A usually short piece of written work that focuses on a topic.
13. To make a product.
14. To come up with.

DOWN

1. To tell as different.
2. The main point of the story or the text; the unifying element of a story or text, sometimes called main idea or theme.
3. Name; identify.
5. An answer or reply.
6. Put together; create.
7. Put in order; put in a series.
8. A group of words within a text.
9. Say; affirm.

A. Predict	B. Sequence	C. Formulate	D. Response	E. Distinguish
F. Formulate	G. Revision	H. Phrase	I. Compare	J. Create
K. Diagram	L. Label	M. Central idea	N. Passage	O. Narrative
P. Sort	Q. State			

14. *Using the Across and Down clues, write the correct words in the numbered grid below.*

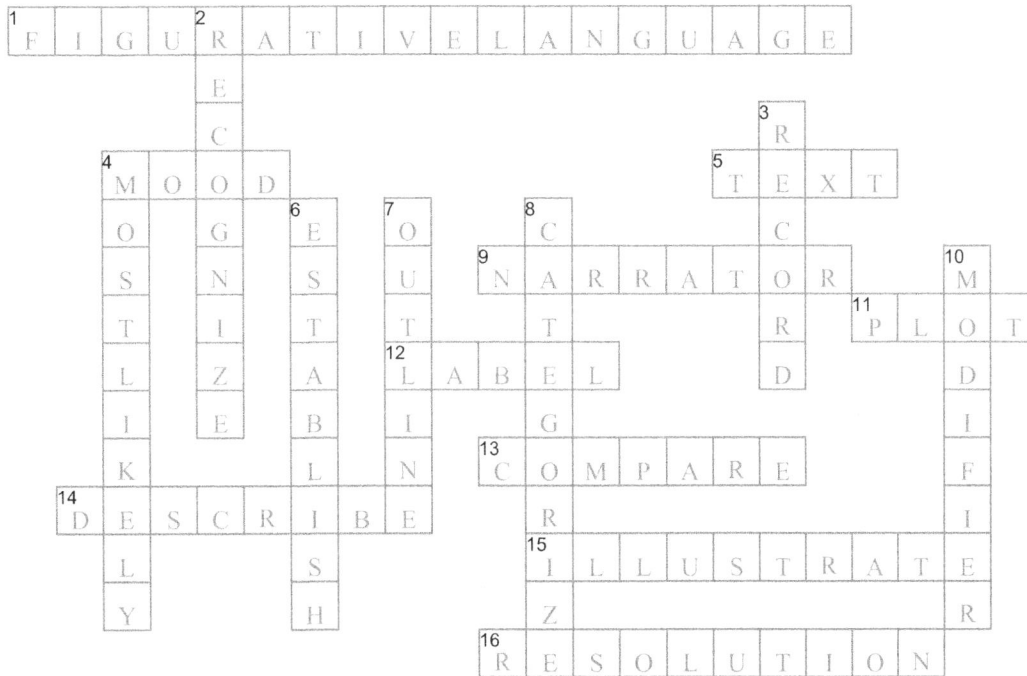

¹F	I	G	U	²R	A	T	I	V	E	L	A	N	G	U	A	G	E	

Grid letters (reading):

1 Across: FIGURATIVELANGUAGE
2 Down: RECOGNIZE
4 Down: MOSTLIKELY
4 Across: MOOD
5 Across: TEXT
3 Down: RECORD
6 Down: ESTABLISH
7 Down: OUTLINE
8 Down: CATEGORIZE
9 Across: NARRATOR
11 Across: PLOT
10 Down: MODIFIER
12 Across: LABEL
13 Across: COMPARE
14 Across: DESCRIBE
15 Across: ILLUSTRATE
16 Across: RESOLUTION

ACROSS

1. Words that may not literally mean what they say.
4. A temporary state of mind or feeling.
5. The reading passage.
9. A person who tells something; storyteller.
11. To determine and mark points on a graph.
12. Name; identify.
13. Tell how alike; judge against.
14. To tell or write about something in detail.
15. To make clear by using examples.
16. The ending, answer, or conclusion to a problem or story.

DOWN

2. To identify from knowledge of appearance or characteristics.
3. To put down in writing so that it is saved.
4. Will probably happen; probably.
6. To show to be true, to prove.
7. Give a rough idea; plan.
8. To put in a group based on certain characteristics.
10. A word, phrase or clause used to describe or qualify another word, phrase or clause.

A. Outline
E. Compare
I. Record
M. Categorize
Q. Narrator

B. Label
F. Modifier
J. Establish
N. Text

C. Figurative language
G. Most likely
K. Recognize
O. Illustrate

D. Mood
H. Resolution
L. Describe
P. Plot

15. *Using the Across and Down clues, write the correct words in the numbered grid below.*

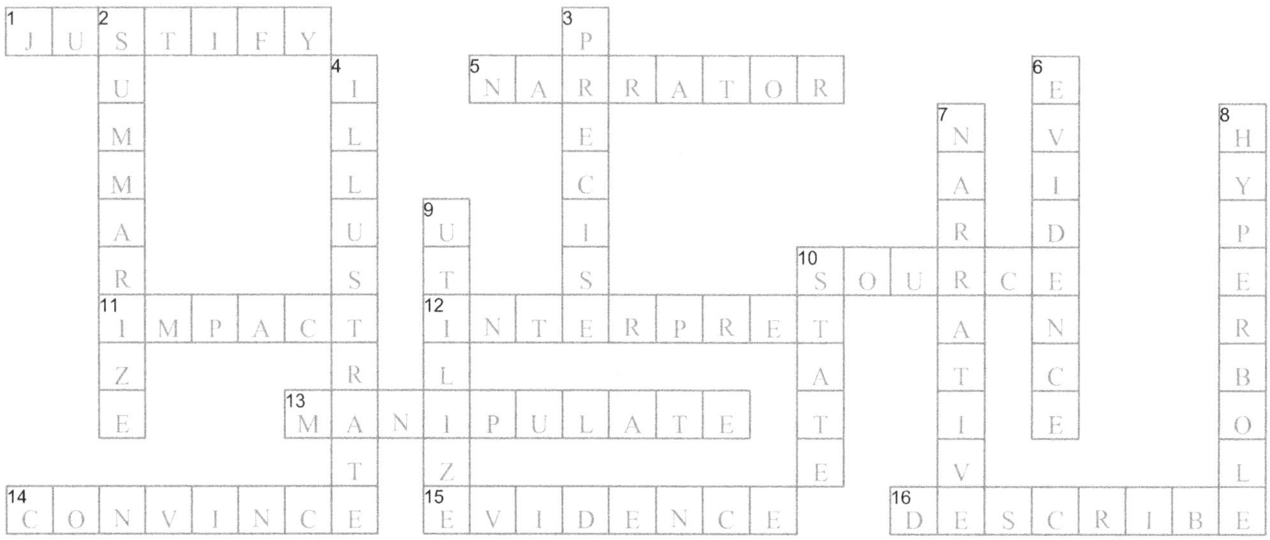

Crossword grid answers:
- 1 Across: JUSTIFY
- 2 Down: SUMMARIZE
- 3 Down: PRECISE
- 4 Down: ILLUSTRATE
- 5 Across: NARRATOR
- 6 Down: EVIDENCE
- 7 Down: NARRATIVE
- 8 Down: HYPERBOLE
- 9 Down: UTILIZE
- 10 Across: SOURCE
- 10 Down: STATE
- 11 Across: IMPACT
- 12 Across: INTERPRET
- 13 Across: MANIPULATE
- 14 Across: CONVINCE
- 15 Across: EVIDENCE
- 16 Across: DESCRIBE

ACROSS

1. To prove.
5. A person who tells something; storyteller.
10. A book, person, or document used to provide information or data.
11. To cause changes.
12. To determine the meaning of.
13. To change something to work in a certain way.
14. To persuade or get someone to think a certain way.
15. Proof; information in the text that proves a point.
16. Tell about; explain.

DOWN

2. Sum it up; give a short version.
3. Exact or specific.
4. To draw or make pictures to explain.
6. Proof; lines and words from text used to prove or disprove an idea.
7. A story.
8. Exaggeration, not meant to be literal.
9. Use something to help find a solution.
10. Say; affirm.

A. Summarize   B. Hyperbole   C. Illustrate   D. Interpret   E. Justify
F. Convince   G. Narrative   H. Utilize   I. Precise   J. Impact
K. Evidence   L. Source   M. Narrator   N. State   O. Evidence
P. Describe   Q. Manipulate

16. *Using the Across and Down clues, write the correct words in the numbered grid below.*

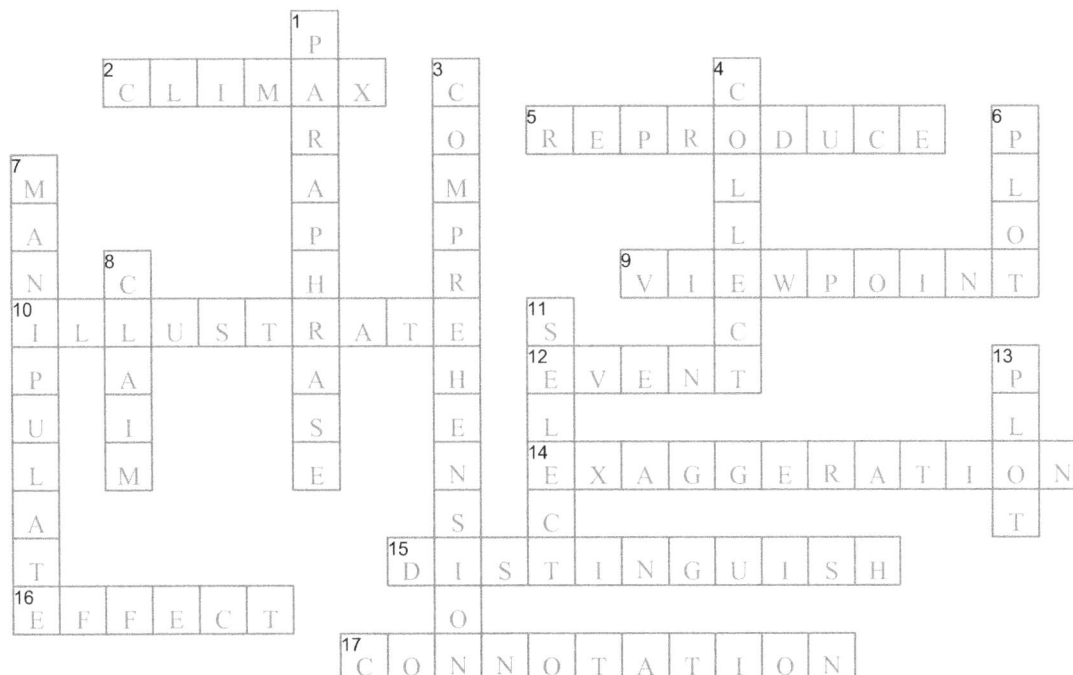

Crossword grid answers:
- 2 Across: CLIMAX
- 5 Across: REPRODUCE
- 9 Across: VIEWPOINT
- 10 Across: ILLUSTRATE
- 12 Across: EVENT
- 14 Across: EXAGGERATION
- 15 Across: DISTINGUISH
- 16 Across: EFFECT
- 17 Across: CONNOTATION
- 1 Down: PARAPHRASE
- 3 Down: COMPREHENSION
- 4 Down: COLLECT
- 6 Down: PLOT
- 7 Down: MANIPULATE
- 8 Down: CLAIM
- 11 Down: SELECT
- 13 Down: PLOT

ACROSS

2. The moment in the story where the conflict reaches its highest point.

5. Copy; repeat.

9. A way of looking or thinking about something.

10. To make clear by using examples.

12. Anything that happens, especially something important or unusual.

14. The fact of making something seem larger, more important, better, or worse than it really is; overstate the truth.

15. To tell as different.

16. What happens because of something.

17. All the meanings, associations, emotions, or tones that a word suggests.

DOWN

1. A restatement of the meaning of a text or passage using other words.

3. The meaning a reader gets from written text.

4. To gather together.

6. To determine and mark points on a graph.

7. To change something to work in a certain way.

8. To state a position or declare that something is true or factual, noun-a statement of truth or fact, typically pertaining to an idea that is disputed.

11. To choose.

13. The events that make up the story or the main part of the story. The events relate to each other in a pattern or sequence.

A. Plot
E. Climax
I. Plot
M. Illustrate
Q. Paraphrase

B. Manipulate
F. Distinguish
J. Select
N. Collect

C. Connotation
G. Effect
K. Viewpoint
O. Exaggeration

D. Reproduce
H. Claim
L. Comprehension
P. Event

17. *Using the Across and Down clues, write the correct words in the numbered grid below.*

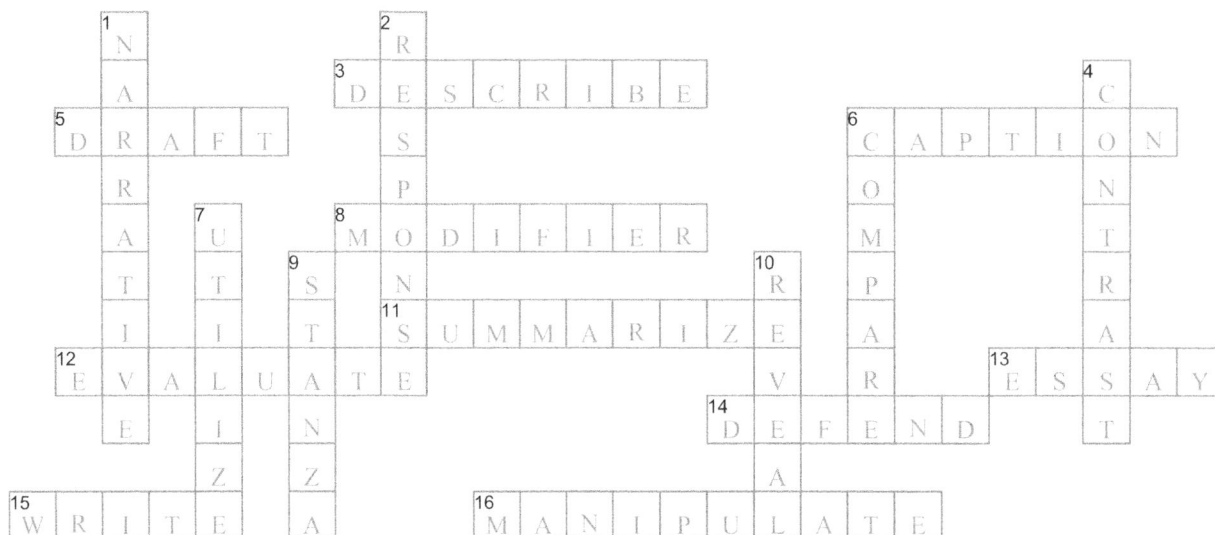

Grid answers:
- 3 Across: DESCRIBE
- 5 Across: DRAFT
- 6 Across: CAPTION
- 8 Across: MODIFIER
- 11 Across: SUMMARIZE
- 12 Across: EVALUATE
- 13 Across: ESSAY
- 14 Across: DEFEND
- 15 Across: WRITE A
- 16 Across: MANIPULATE
- 1 Down: NARRATIVE
- 2 Down: RESPONSE
- 4 Down: CONTRAST
- 6 Down: COMPARE
- 7 Down: UTILIZE
- 9 Down: STANZA
- 10 Down: REVEAL

ACROSS

3. To tell or write about something in detail.

5. Plain; rough copy.

6. An explanation for a picture or illustration.

8. A word, phrase or clause used to describe or qualify another word, phrase or clause.

11. Sum it up; give a short version.

12. Judge; consider.

13. A short literary composition on a theme or subject - usually analytic or interpretive in nature.

14. Support; uphold.

15. To produce words.

16. To change something to work in a certain way.

DOWN

1. A story.

2. An answer or reply.

4. To find differences.

6. Explain how things are the same.

7. Use something to help find a solution.

9. A group of lines forming the basic unit in a poem; a verse.

10. To show or make known.

A. Modifier   B. Evaluate   C. Describe   D. Compare   E. Contrast
F. Essay   G. Manipulate   H. Caption   I. Response   J. Write
K. Stanza   L. Narrative   M. Reveal   N. Summarize   O. Draft
P. Utilize   Q. Defend

18. *Using the Across and Down clues, write the correct words in the numbered grid below.*

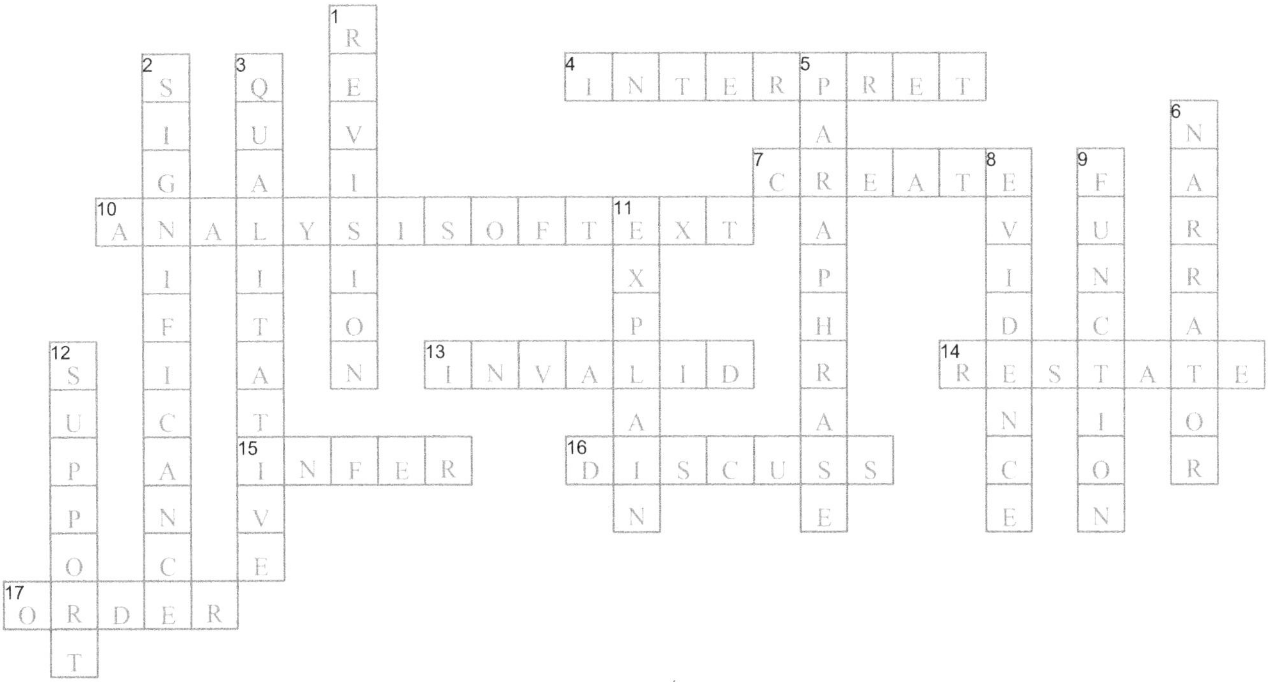

ACROSS

4. Explain the meaning; make clear.
7. To make a product.
10. Read and examine text in detail looking for important ideas.
13. Not true.
14. Repeat; say again.
15. Make a good guess; read between the lines.
16. Talk about; argue.
17. Sort; organize.

DOWN

1. A corrected or new version of something written.
2. A part of the story that is important.
3. Data that is based on numbers.
5. A restatement of the meaning of a text or passage using other words.
6. A person who tells something; storyteller.
8. Proof; information in the text that proves a point.
9. Job, what it does.
11. Make clear; put in your own words.
12. To provide proof or evidence for.

A. Significance
B. Invalid
C. Paraphrase
D. Explain
E. Analysis of text
F. Function
G. Revision
H. Evidence
I. Narrator
J. Support
K. Order
L. Interpret
M. Discuss
N. Create
O. Qualitative
P. Restate
Q. Infer

19. *Using the Across and Down clues, write the correct words in the numbered grid below.*

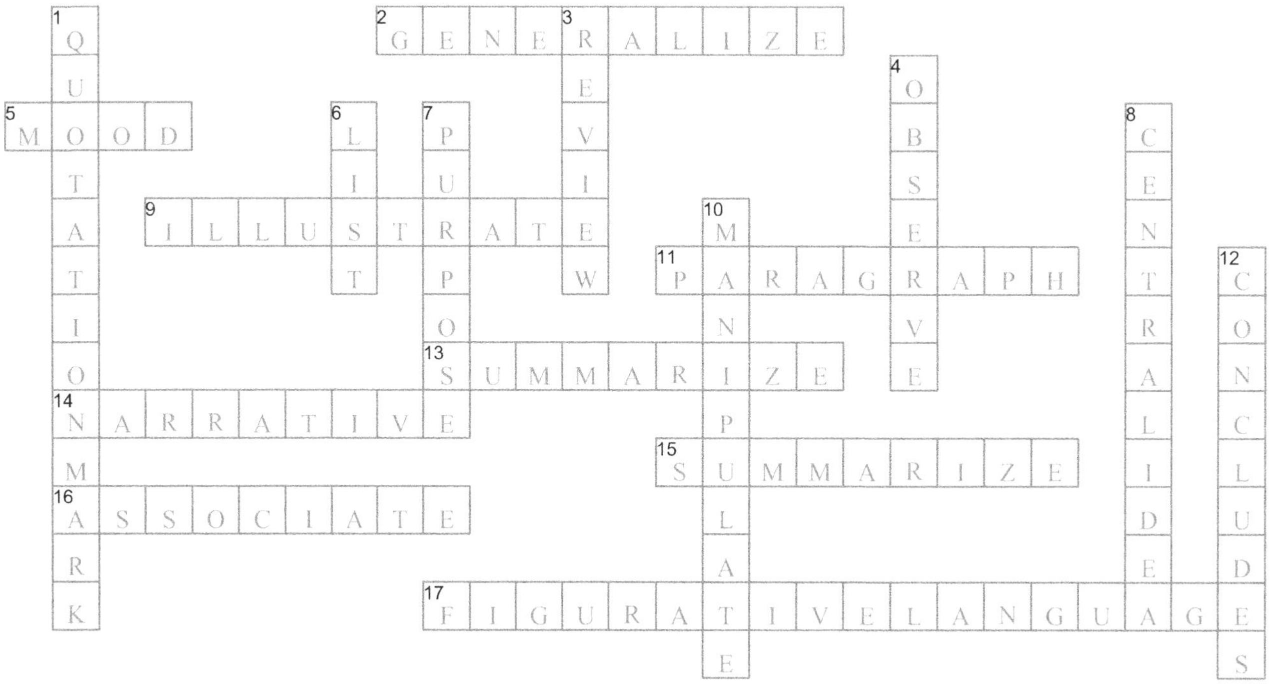

1 QUOTATION MARK
2 GENERALIZE
3 REVIEW
4 OBSERVE
5 MOOD
6 LIST
7 PURPOSE
8 CENTRAL IDEA
9 ILLUSTRATE
10 MANIPULATE
11 PARAGRAPH
12 CONCLUDES
13 SUMMARIZE
14 NARRATIVE
15 SUMMARIZE
16 ASSOCIATE
17 FIGURATIVE LANGUAGE

ACROSS

2. to make a statement based upon details from the reading passage that might be true in other situations.
5. A temporary state of mind or feeling.
9. To draw or make pictures to explain.
11. A section of writing consisting of one or more sentences grouped together and discussing one main subject.
13. To paraphrase or to explain in your own words an important idea or section of text.
14. A story.
15. Sum it up; give a short version.
16. To relate to concepts.
17. Words or expression different from literal language, changed or altered to make a linguistic point.

DOWN

1. A punctuation mark ", " or ',' used at the beginning and ending of text that has been stated from a source.
3. Look at; study.
4. Watch; notice.
6. Record; name.
7. The reason someone does something.
8. The main point of the story or the text; the unifying element of a story or text, sometimes called main idea or theme.
10. To change something to work in a certain way.
12. To think about carefully and form an opinion.

A. Narrative	B. List	C. Generalize	D. Central idea
E. Paragraph	F. Manipulate	G. Observe	H. Associate
I. Purpose	J. Summarize	K. Summarize	L. Mood
M. Concludes	N. Illustrate	O. Review	P. Figurative language
Q. Quotation mark			

20. *Using the Across and Down clues, write the correct words in the numbered grid below.*

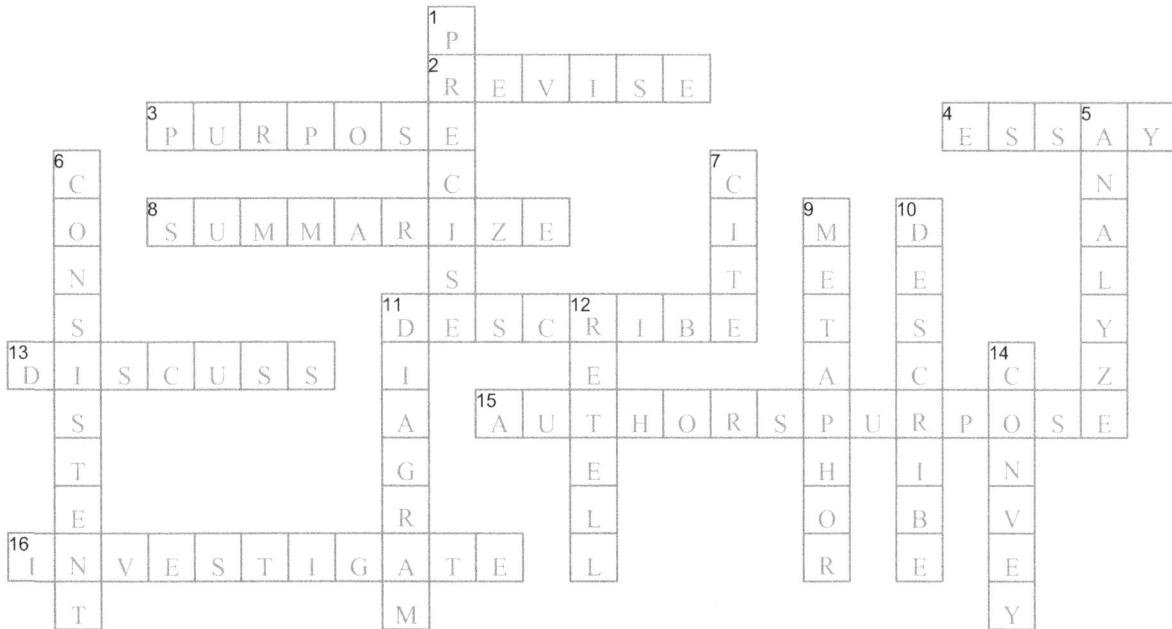

The completed crossword grid contains:
- 2 Across: REVISE
- 3 Across: PURPOSE
- 4 Across: ESSAY
- 8 Across: SUMMARIZE
- 11 Across: DESCRIBE
- 13 Across: DISCUSS
- 15 Across: AUTHORSPURPOSE
- 16 Across: INVESTIGATE
- 1 Down: PRECISE
- 5 Down: ANALYZE
- 6 Down: CONSISTE (CONSISTENT)
- 7 Down: CITE
- 9 Down: METAPHOR
- 10 Down: DESCRIBE
- 11 Down: DIAGRAM
- 12 Down: REELL (RETELL)
- 14 Down: CONVEY

ACROSS

2. Change; alter.

3. The reason someone does something.

4. A short literary composition on a theme or subject - usually analytic or interpretive in nature.

8. Sum it up; give a short version.

11. Tell about; explain.

13. To consider an idea.

15. Reason the author writes: persuade, inform, entertain (PIE).

16. To search for an answer to a solution.

DOWN

1. Exact or specific.

5. Break apart; study the pieces.

6. To do something the same constantly.

7. To use a quote from the text to support an idea.

9. A comparison of two unlike things by describing one is the other.

10. To tell or write about something in detail.

11. A simplified drawing.

12. Repeat; say again.

14. To make things or ideas known to others; to share or to get ideas across to others.

A. Metaphor   B. Precise   C. Convey   D. Revise
E. Authors purpose   F. Discuss   G. Summarize   H. Analyze
I. Diagram   J. Describe   K. Retell   L. Describe
M. Investigate   N. Purpose   O. Essay   P. Consistent
Q. Cite

Multiple Choice

From the words provided for each clue, provide the letter of the word which best matches the clue.

1. __ A conclusion reached based on reasoning and the use of given facts; a prediction.
   A.Compare B.Simile C.Inference D.Interpret

2. __ A single piece of information or fact about something.
   A.Character B.Summarize C.Detail D.Select

3. __ To make clear by using examples.
   A.Illustrate B.Defend C.Interpret D.Explain

4. __ Proof; lines and words from text used to prove or disprove an idea.
   A.Evidence B.Central idea C.Response D.Text

5. __ Judge; consider.
   A.Diagram B.Attitude C.Evaluate D.Retell

6. __ Label the parts of the drawing; make a drawing, chart, or plan.
   A.Cause B.Diagram C.Conclude D.Categorize

7. __ To prove.
   A.Text B.Defend C.Precise D.Justify

8. __ Job, what it does.
   A.Contrast B.Justify C.Function D.Character

9. __ A comparison of two unlike things using the words "like" or "as".
   A.Revision B.Plot C.Simile D.Restate

10. __ A corrected or new version of something written.
    A.Assess B.Revision C.Text D.Authors purpose

11. __ To tell or write about something in detail.
    A.Label B.Identify C.Describe D.Cause

12. __ Clearly express something in a speech or writing.
    A.State B.Infer C.Cause D.Best

13. __ Exact or specific.
    A.Analysis of text B.Develop C.Precise D.Draft

14. __ Copy; repeat.
    A.Reproduce B.Describe C.Evaluate D.Phrase

15. __ The main point of the story or the text; the unifying element of a story or text, sometimes called main idea or theme.
    A.Reveal B.Plot C.Restate D.Central idea

16. __ Give an instance; case.
    A.Example B.Calculate C.Select D.Italics

17. __ A group of words within a text.
    A.Phrase B.Explain C.Suspense D.Simile

18. __ Finish; end.
A.Enclosed B.Complete C.Detail D.Evidence

19. __ Look at; inspect.
A.Simile B.Establish C.Plot D.Examine

20. __ What the passage or text is mainly about.
A.Central idea B.Define C.Topic D.Caption

21. __ Make a good guess; read between the lines.
A.Infer B.Create C.Collect D.Establish

22. __ To state a position or declare that something is true or factual, noun-a statement of truth or fact, typically pertaining to an idea that is disputed.
A.Select B.Claim C.Text D.Evidence

23. __ A usually short piece of written work that focuses on a topic.
A.Complete B.Justify C.Evaluate D.Passage

24. __ Text that the author presents as an argument.
A.Reveal B.Textual evidence C.Contrast D.Best

25. __ Repeat; say again.
A.Result B.Retell C.Exaggeration D.Enclosed

26. __ What happens because of something.
A.Suspense B.Effect C.Character D.Best

27. __ Ending; wrapping up.
A.Claim B.Conclusion C.Passage D.Explain

28. __ Proof; information in the text that proves a point.
A.Evidence B.Outline C.Denotation D.Decode

29. __ Helps to support the central idea in an important way. Authors elaborate using examples or anecdotes.
A.Best B.Key detail C.Suspense D.Conclude

30. __ A short literary composition on a theme or subject - usually analytic or interpretive in nature.
A.Contrast B.Essay C.Model D.Excerpt

31. __ To represent something that will serve as an example.
A.Revision B.Explain C.Character D.Model

32. __ Tell how things are different; draw a distinction.
A.Example B.Contrast C.Paragraph D.Summarize

33. __ Make clear; put in your own words.
A.Effective B.Explain C.Character D.Example

34. __ Describe; characterize.
A.Define B.Excerpt C.Topic D.Key detail

35. __ A style of print where the letters slope to the right; may be used to emphasize or to indicate the title of published work.
A.Invalid B.Italics C.Model D.Topic

36. __ Name; identify.
A.Revision B.Text C.Classify D.Label

37. __ A part of a reading passage.
A.Topic B.Classify C.Excerpt D.Effect

38. __ Make out; break apart.
A.Decode B.Effective C.State D.Collect

39. __ Exaggeration, not meant to be literal.
A.Caption B.Convey C.Event D.Hyperbole

40. __ Above all others, most desirable.
A.Explain B.Character C.Best D.Select

41. __ To choose.
A.Response B.Select C.Authors purpose D.Revise

42. __ The way someone feels about something.
A.Attitude B.Interpret C.Utilize D.Revision

43. __ Explain the meaning; make clear.
A.Cite B.Interpret C.Detail D.Essay

44. __ The events that make up the story or the main part of the story. The events relate to each other in a pattern or sequence.
A.Plot B.Sequence C.Effect D.Examine

45. __ Able to do its job to the best ability.
A.Classify B.Construct C.Effective D.Complete

46. __ To determine and mark points on a graph.
A.Claim B.Plot C.Response D.Evaluate

47. __ To gather together.
A.Justify B.Interpret C.Collect D.Classify

48. __ The way a text is presented: introduction, headings and
A.Best B.Utilize C.Justify D.Text structure

49. __ A story.
A.Develop B.Describe C.Narrative D.Claim

50. __ Put in order; put in a series.
A.Model B.Establish C.Plot D.Sequence

51. __ To make a product.
A.Utilize B.Narrative C.Simile D.Create

52. __ to decide based upon information stated in the reading passages.
A.Establish B.Conclusion C.Conclude D.Describe

53. __ Judge; consider.
   A.Assess B.Paragraph C.Analysis of text D.Calculate

54. __ Put in order; sort.
   A.Contrast B.Compare C.Function D.Classify

55. __ To draw or make pictures to explain.
   A.Function B.Evidence C.Illustrate D.Determine

56. __ Anything that happens, especially something important or unusual.
   A.Infer B.Event C.Examine D.Evidence

57. __ Repeat; say again.
   A.Restate B.Revise C.Complete D.Construct

58. __ To connect back to another text.
   A.Define B.Reference C.Draft D.Illustrate

59. __ To use a quote from the text to support an idea.
   A.Interpret B.Cite C.Outline D.Evidence

60. __ Read and examine text in detail looking for important ideas.
   A.Develop B.Analysis of text C.Narrative D.Phrase

61. __ Tell about; explain.
   A.Caption B.Cite C.Key detail D.Describe

62. __ To give details to make something clear.
   A.Explain B.Attitude C.Complete D.Label

63. __ Not sure what is going to happen, waiting.
   A.Outline B.Suspense C.Inference D.Explain

64. __ A section of writing consisting of one or more sentences grouped together and discussing one main subject.
   A.Identify B.Paragraph C.Plot D.Evidence

65. __ To recognize or establish as being a person or thing.
   A.Identify B.Figurative language C.Plot D.Label

66. __ To work out, grow, or expand.
   A.Topic B.Evidence C.Develop D.Event

67. __ To paraphrase or to explain in your own words an important idea or section of text.
   A.Summarize B.Select C.Hyperbole D.Text

68. __ An answer or reply.
   A.Sequence B.Illustrate C.Reproduce D.Response

69. __ Not true.
   A.Example B.Evidence C.Invalid D.Result

70. __ The subject of discussion or the subject of the article.
   A.Label B.Explain C.Topic D.Define

71. __ To decide.
A.Interpret B.Determine C.Describe D.Outline

72. __ A restatement of the meaning of a text or passage using other words.
A.Paraphrase B.Narrative C.Classify D.Topic

73. __ Change; alter.
A.Summarize B.Revision C.Key detail D.Revise

74. __ The basic definition or dictionary meaning of a word.
A.Paraphrase B.Denotation C.Central idea D.Excerpt

75. __ Give an answer; consequence.
A.Contrast B.Reproduce C.Result D.Key detail

76. __ Words that may not literally mean what they say.
A.Evidence B.Cause C.Figurative language D.Interpret

77. __ Using few words to give the most important information about something or a complete but brief account of things previously stated.
A.Attitude B.Cite C.Summary D.Draft

78. __ An explanation for a picture or illustration.
A.Caption B.Function C.Summarize D.Interpret

79. __ Support; uphold.
A.Revision B.Central idea C.Result D.Defend

80. __ The reason why something happens.
A.Plot B.Function C.Effect D.Cause

81. __ Sort; organize.
A.Event B.Order C.Text D.Hyperbole

82. __ Reason the author writes: persuade, inform, entertain (PIE).
A.Diagram B.Italics C.Authors purpose D.Result

83. __ Use something to help find a solution.
A.Develop B.Claim C.Diagram D.Utilize

84. __ To use.
A.Select B.Apply C.Plot D.Decode

85. __ To make things or ideas known to others; to share or to get ideas across to others.
A.Convey B.Detail C.Claim D.Evidence

86. __ Explain how things are different.
A.Complete B.Contrast C.Text D.Claim

87. __ Work out; compute.
A.Calculate B.Summary C.Draft D.Narrative

88. __ Plain; rough copy.
A.Infer B.Result C.Draft D.Narrative

89. __ To show to be true, to prove.
A.Establish B.Contrast C.Text structure D.Evidence

90. __ A person in a novel, play, or movie or any person, animal or figure represented in a literary work.
A.Best B.Character C.Outline D.Cause

91. __ Give a rough idea; plan.
A.Evidence B.Outline C.Conclude D.Summarize

92. __ The fact of making something seem larger, more important, better, or worse than it really is; overstate the truth.
A.Paragraph B.Authors purpose C.Order D.Exaggeration

93. __ To show or make known.
A.Function B.Classify C.Reveal D.Calculate

94. __ To make a product.
A.Construct B.Cite C.Explain D.Effective

95. __ To find similarities.
A.Complete B.Sequence C.Categorize D.Compare

96. __ To include with something else (e.g. the money is enclosed with the letter in the envelope); to close or hold in.
A.Calculate B.Best C.Summary D.Enclosed

97. __ A simplified drawing.
A.Reference B.Diagram C.Example D.Draft

98. __ To put in a group based on certain characteristics.
A.Categorize B.Analysis of text C.Response D.Decode

99. __ To determine the meaning of.
A.Examine B.Interpret C.Retell D.Justify

100. __ The reading passage.
A.Text B.Evidence C.Result D.Model

From the words provided for each clue, provide the letter of the word which best matches the clue.

101. __ To make a product.
A.Inference B.Collect C.Create D.Assess

102. __ To gather together.
A.State B.Infer C.Most likely D.Collect

103. __ Put in order; arrange.
A.Organize B.Convince C.Contribute D.Analysis of text

104. __ To persuade or get someone to think a certain way.
A.Support B.Convince C.Narrative D.Imply

105. __ What happens because of something.
A.Mood B.Effect C.Suspense D.Result

106. __ Name; label.
A.Identify B.Analyze C.Evidence D.Infer

107. __ To merge two or more sentences into one sentence.
A.Effect B.Combine sentences C.Paraphrase D.Contrast

108. __ The events that make up the story or the main part of the story. The events relate to each other in a pattern or sequence.
A.Plot B.Assess C.Evidence D.Denotation

109. __ A comparison of two unlike things using the words "like" or "as".
A.Explain B.Result C.Infer D.Simile

110. __ What one thinks about something or somebody.
A.Create B.Opinion C.Establish D.Denotation

111. __ To make clear by using examples.
A.Resolution B.Illustrate C.Hyperbole D.Support

112. __ To produce words.
A.Discuss B.Infer C.Write D.Connotation

113. __ To use a quote from the text to support an idea.
A.Topic B.Describe C.Write D.Cite

114. __ Data that uses characteristics.
A.Justify B.Identify C.Quantitative D.Support

115. __ What the passage or text is mainly about.
A.Impact B.Narrative C.Perspective D.Central idea

116. __ Give good reason; defend.
A.Discuss B.Suspense C.Claim D.Justify

117. __ A part of the story that is important.
A.Significance B.State C.Support D.Outline

118. __ Reason the author writes: persuade, inform, entertain (PIE).
A.Convey B.Authors purpose C.Organize D.Response

119. __ An opinion or the way someone looks at something.
A.Best B.Select C.Perspective D.Qualitative

120. __ Exaggeration, not meant to be literal.
A.Interpret B.Hyperbole C.Review D.Distinguish

121. __ To make known in detail.
A.Explain B.Define C.Outline D.Examine

122. __ Copy; repeat.
A.Reproduce B.Analysis of text C.Calculate D.Text

123. __ To choose.
A.Combine sentences   B.Support   C.Central idea   D.Select

124. __ To make a product.
A.Construct   B.Combine sentences   C.Key detail   D.Most likely

125. __ The reason why something happens.
A.Contrast   B.Collect   C.Cause   D.Caption

126. __ Work out; compute.
A.Observe   B.Calculate   C.Demonstrate   D.Viewpoint

127. __ A part of a reading passage.
A.Excerpt   B.Justify   C.Figurative language   D.Sequence

128. __ Sum it up; give a short version.
A.Qualitative   B.Summarize   C.Complete   D.Convince

129. __ The reading passage.
A.Text   B.Support   C.Establish   D.Review

130. __ A way of looking or thinking about something.
A.Viewpoint   B.Hyperbole   C.State   D.Illustrate

131. __ Ending; wrapping up.
A.Conclusion   B.Describe   C.Purpose   D.Key detail

132. __ To provide proof or evidence for.
A.Purpose   B.Support   C.Calculate   D.Narrative

133. __ To put down in writing so that it is saved.
A.Figurative language   B.Text   C.Record   D.Analyze

134. __ Make a good guess; read between the lines.
A.Key detail   B.Illustrate   C.Infer   D.Review

135. __ The ending, answer, or conclusion to a problem or story.
A.Resolution   B.Infer   C.Inference   D.Interpret

136. __ To state a position or declare that something is true or factual, noun-a statement of truth or fact, typically pertaining to an idea that is disputed.
A.Illustrate   B.Narrative   C.Explain   D.Claim

137. __ To show to be true, to prove.
A.Effect   B.Establish   C.Calculate   D.Construct

138. __ A conclusion reached based on reasoning and the use of given facts; a prediction.
A.Concludes   B.Central idea   C.Inference   D.Valid

139. __ A comparison of two unlike things by describing one is the other.
A.Metaphor   B.Explain   C.Caption   D.Interpret

140. __ Give an answer; consequence.
A.Contrast   B.Result   C.Sequence   D.Construct

141. __ To tell the facts, details.
      A.Contrast B.Support C.Illustrate D.Describe

142. __ Using few words to give the most important information about something or a complete
      but brief account of things previously stated.
      A.Authors purpose B.Tone C.State D.Summary

143. __ A book or other written work or printed work.
      A.Distinguish B.Effect C.Text D.Suspense

144. __ Look at; study.
      A.Illustrate B.Imply C.Response D.Review

145. __ Give a rough idea; plan.
      A.Describe B.Interpret C.Outline D.Narrative

146. __ A punctuation mark ", " or ',' used at the beginning and ending of text that has been stated
      from a source.
      A.Describe B.Support C.Examine D.Quotation mark

147. __ Use details from the text to explain your response.
      A.Connotation B.Summary C.Construct D.Support

148. __ Proof; lines and words from text used to prove or disprove an idea.
      A.Denotation B.Demonstrate C.Stanza D.Evidence

149. __ to hint at something without saying it.
      A.Imply B.Demonstrate C.Plot D.Identify

150. __ The subject of discussion or the subject of the article.
      A.Effect B.Convey C.Topic D.Convince

151. __ To look at text carefully by paying attention to its parts, its words, its figurative language,
      and its tone.
      A.Demonstrate B.Analysis of text C.Analyze D.Resolution

152. __ Tell about; explain.
      A.Convey B.Sequence C.Summarize D.Describe

153. __ To determine the meaning of.
      A.Plot B.Interpret C.Hyperbole D.Tone

154. __ Talk about; argue.
      A.Defend B.Discuss C.Illustrate D.Sequence

155. __ Above all others, most desirable.
      A.Quotation mark B.Simile C.Best D.Discuss

156. __ Look at; inspect.
      A.Summarize B.Examine C.Effect D.Cite

157. __ Describe; characterize.
      A.Collect B.Most likely C.Plot D.Define

158. __ Not sure what is going to happen, waiting.
A.Suspense B.Combine sentences C.Figurative language D.Contrast

159. __ Words or expression different from literal language, changed or altered to make a linguistic point.
A.Construct B.Simile C.Impact D.Figurative language

160. __ The basic definition or dictionary meaning of a word.
A.Valid B.Cite C.Denotation D.Write

161. __ Read and examine text in detail looking for important ideas.
A.Analysis of text B.Create C.Most likely D.Contribute

162. __ A temporary state of mind or feeling.
A.Central idea B.Opinion C.Mood D.Establish

163. __ Put in order; put in a series.
A.Cause B.Sequence C.Authors purpose D.Reveal

164. __ Say; affirm.
A.Claim B.State C.Quotation mark D.Plot

165. __ A restatement of the meaning of a text or passage using other words.
A.Paraphrase B.Describe C.Cite D.Analysis of text

166. __ To paraphrase or to explain in your own words an important idea or section of text.
A.Mood B.Summarize C.Explain D.Result

167. __ An explanation for a picture or illustration.
A.Denotation B.Distinguish C.Caption D.Response

168. __ Support; uphold.
A.Perspective B.Interpret C.Evidence D.Defend

169. __ Helps to support the central idea in an important way. Authors elaborate using examples or anecdotes.
A.Discuss B.Key detail C.Convince D.Effect

170. __ To cause changes.
A.Impact B.Perspective C.Paraphrase D.Excerpt

171. __ An answer or reply.
A.Caption B.Central idea C.Response D.Simile

172. __ A story.
A.Qualitative B.Authors purpose C.Quantitative D.Narrative

173. __ To make things or ideas known to others; to share or to get ideas across to others.
A.Mood B.Perspective C.Convey D.Organize

174. __ To show or make known.
A.Reveal B.Result C.Convince D.Effective

175. __ To consider an idea.
A.Cite B.Discuss C.Establish D.Convey

176. __ All the meanings, associations, emotions, or tones that a word suggests.
A.Distinguish B.Observe C.Connotation D.Narrative

177. __ To judge or determine the quality or amount of something.
A.Illustrate B.Evaluate C.Perspective D.Conclusion

178. __ Data that is based on numbers.
A.Interpret B.Authors purpose C.Qualitative D.Collect

179. __ Sort; organize.
A.Order B.Justify C.Support D.Convey

180. __ Proof; information in the text that proves a point.
A.Combine sentences B.Viewpoint C.Central idea D.Evidence

181. __ True.
A.Review B.Valid C.Explain D.Discuss

182. __ Give the facts; back up with details.
A.Mood B.Describe C.Excerpt D.Support

183. __ To find differences.
A.Observe B.Central idea C.Contrast D.Infer

184. __ The main point of the story or the text; the unifying element of a story or text, sometimes called main idea or theme.
A.Create B.Central idea C.Reproduce D.Contribute

185. __ Judge; consider.
A.Define B.Support C.Assess D.Cite

186. __ Will probably happen; probably.
A.Plot B.Combine sentences C.Justify D.Most likely

187. __ Able to do its job to the best ability.
A.Best B.Record C.Identify D.Effective

188. __ Show; make plain.
A.Demonstrate B.Tone C.Key detail D.Simile

189. __ A writer's attitude toward his or her topic which is revealed through specific words used in the text and through figurative language.
A.Support B.Tone C.Concludes D.Paraphrase

190. __ To tell or write about something in detail.
A.Describe B.Support C.Quotation mark D.Sequence

191. __ To think about carefully and form an opinion.
A.Concludes B.Resolution C.Support D.Infer

192. __ To help happen or help cause.
A.Contrast B.Contribute C.Illustrate D.Infer

193. __ Finish; end.
A.Complete B.Summarize C.Quotation mark D.Connotation

194. __ Make clear; put in your own words.
    A.Central idea   B.Explain   C.Figurative language   D.Inference

195. __ A group of lines in a poem (similar to a paragraph).
    A.Opinion   B.Infer   C.Stanza   D.Perspective

196. __ To draw or make pictures to explain.
    A.Central idea   B.Describe   C.Excerpt   D.Illustrate

197. __ To explain an idea or make a conclusion by looking closely at evidence in text.
    A.Summarize   B.Key detail   C.Infer   D.Discuss

198. __ The reason someone does something.
    A.Purpose   B.Demonstrate   C.Connotation   D.Collect

199. __ Watch; notice.
    A.Observe   B.Examine   C.Most likely   D.Metaphor

200. __ To tell as different.
    A.Distinguish   B.Conclusion   C.Connotation   D.Establish

From the words provided for each clue, provide the letter of the word which best matches the clue.

1. C A conclusion reached based on reasoning and the use of given facts; a prediction.
   A.Compare B.Simile C.Inference D.Interpret

2. C A single piece of information or fact about something.
   A.Character B.Summarize C.Detail D.Select

3. A To make clear by using examples.
   A.Illustrate B.Defend C.Interpret D.Explain

4. A Proof; lines and words from text used to prove or disprove an idea.
   A.Evidence B.Central idea C.Response D.Text

5. C Judge; consider.
   A.Diagram B.Attitude C.Evaluate D.Retell

6. B Label the parts of the drawing; make a drawing, chart, or plan.
   A.Cause B.Diagram C.Conclude D.Categorize

7. D To prove.
   A.Text B.Defend C.Precise D.Justify

8. C Job, what it does.
   A.Contrast B.Justify C.Function D.Character

9. C A comparison of two unlike things using the words "like" or "as".
   A.Revision B.Plot C.Simile D.Restate

10. B A corrected or new version of something written.
    A.Assess B.Revision C.Text D.Authors purpose

11. C To tell or write about something in detail.
    A.Label B.Identify C.Describe D.Cause

12. A Clearly express something in a speech or writing.
    A.State B.Infer C.Cause D.Best

13. C Exact or specific.
    A.Analysis of text B.Develop C.Precise D.Draft

14. A Copy; repeat.
    A.Reproduce B.Describe C.Evaluate D.Phrase

15. D The main point of the story or the text; the unifying element of a story or text, sometimes called main idea or theme.
    A.Reveal B.Plot C.Restate D.Central idea

16. A Give an instance; case.
    A.Example B.Calculate C.Select D.Italics

17. A A group of words within a text.
    A.Phrase B.Explain C.Suspense D.Simile

18. B Finish; end.
    A.Enclosed B.Complete C.Detail D.Evidence

19. D Look at; inspect.
    A.Simile B.Establish C.Plot D.Examine

20. A What the passage or text is mainly about.
    A.Central idea B.Define C.Topic D.Caption

21. A Make a good guess; read between the lines.
    A.Infer B.Create C.Collect D.Establish

22. B To state a position or declare that something is true or factual, noun-a statement of truth or fact, typically pertaining to an idea that is disputed.
    A.Select B.Claim C.Text D.Evidence

23. D A usually short piece of written work that focuses on a topic.
    A.Complete B.Justify C.Evaluate D.Passage

24. B Text that the author presents as an argument.
    A.Reveal B.Textual evidence C.Contrast D.Best

25. B Repeat; say again.
    A.Result B.Retell C.Exaggeration D.Enclosed

26. B What happens because of something.
    A.Suspense B.Effect C.Character D.Best

27. B Ending; wrapping up.
    A.Claim B.Conclusion C.Passage D.Explain

28. A Proof; information in the text that proves a point.
    A.Evidence B.Outline C.Denotation D.Decode

29. B Helps to support the central idea in an important way. Authors elaborate using examples or anecdotes.
    A.Best B.Key detail C.Suspense D.Conclude

30. B A short literary composition on a theme or subject - usually analytic or interpretive in nature.
    A.Contrast B.Essay C.Model D.Excerpt

31. D To represent something that will serve as an example.
    A.Revision B.Explain C.Character D.Model

32. B Tell how things are different; draw a distinction.
    A.Example B.Contrast C.Paragraph D.Summarize

33. B Make clear; put in your own words.
    A.Effective B.Explain C.Character D.Example

34. A Describe; characterize.
    A.Define B.Excerpt C.Topic D.Key detail

35. _B_ A style of print where the letters slope to the right; may be used to emphasize or to indicate the title of published work.
A.Invalid B.Italics C.Model D.Topic

36. _D_ Name; identify.
A.Revision B.Text C.Classify D.Label

37. _C_ A part of a reading passage.
A.Topic B.Classify C.Excerpt D.Effect

38. _A_ Make out; break apart.
A.Decode B.Effective C.State D.Collect

39. _D_ Exaggeration, not meant to be literal.
A.Caption B.Convey C.Event D.Hyperbole

40. _C_ Above all others, most desirable.
A.Explain B.Character C.Best D.Select

41. _B_ To choose.
A.Response B.Select C.Authors purpose D.Revise

42. _A_ The way someone feels about something.
A.Attitude B.Interpret C.Utilize D.Revision

43. _B_ Explain the meaning; make clear.
A.Cite B.Interpret C.Detail D.Essay

44. _A_ The events that make up the story or the main part of the story. The events relate to each other in a pattern or sequence.
A.Plot B.Sequence C.Effect D.Examine

45. _C_ Able to do its job to the best ability.
A.Classify B.Construct C.Effective D.Complete

46. _B_ To determine and mark points on a graph.
A.Claim B.Plot C.Response D.Evaluate

47. _C_ To gather together.
A.Justify B.Interpret C.Collect D.Classify

48. _D_ The way a text is presented: introduction, headings and
A.Best B.Utilize C.Justify D.Text structure

49. _C_ A story.
A.Develop B.Describe C.Narrative D.Claim

50. _D_ Put in order; put in a series.
A.Model B.Establish C.Plot D.Sequence

51. _D_ To make a product.
A.Utilize B.Narrative C.Simile D.Create

52. _C_ to decide based upon information stated in the reading passages.
A.Establish B.Conclusion C.Conclude D.Describe

53. A   Judge; consider.
   A.Assess B.Paragraph C.Analysis of text D.Calculate

54. D   Put in order; sort.
   A.Contrast B.Compare C.Function D.Classify

55. C   To draw or make pictures to explain.
   A.Function B.Evidence C.Illustrate D.Determine

56. B   Anything that happens, especially something important or unusual.
   A.Infer B.Event C.Examine D.Evidence

57. A   Repeat; say again.
   A.Restate B.Revise C.Complete D.Construct

58. B   To connect back to another text.
   A.Define B.Reference C.Draft D.Illustrate

59. B   To use a quote from the text to support an idea.
   A.Interpret B.Cite C.Outline D.Evidence

60. B   Read and examine text in detail looking for important ideas.
   A.Develop B.Analysis of text C.Narrative D.Phrase

61. D   Tell about; explain.
   A.Caption B.Cite C.Key detail D.Describe

62. A   To give details to make something clear.
   A.Explain B.Attitude C.Complete D.Label

63. B   Not sure what is going to happen, waiting.
   A.Outline B.Suspense C.Inference D.Explain

64. B   A section of writing consisting of one or more sentences grouped together and discussing one main subject.
   A.Identify B.Paragraph C.Plot D.Evidence

65. A   To recognize or establish as being a person or thing.
   A.Identify B.Figurative language C.Plot D.Label

66. C   To work out, grow, or expand.
   A.Topic B.Evidence C.Develop D.Event

67. A   To paraphrase or to explain in your own words an important idea or section of text.
   A.Summarize B.Select C.Hyperbole D.Text

68. D   An answer or reply.
   A.Sequence B.Illustrate C.Reproduce D.Response

69. C   Not true.
   A.Example B.Evidence C.Invalid D.Result

70. C   The subject of discussion or the subject of the article.
   A.Label B.Explain C.Topic D.Define

71. B   To decide.
    A.Interpret   B.Determine   C.Describe   D.Outline

72. A   A restatement of the meaning of a text or passage using other words.
    A.Paraphrase   B.Narrative   C.Classify   D.Topic

73. D   Change; alter.
    A.Summarize   B.Revision   C.Key detail   D.Revise

74. B   The basic definition or dictionary meaning of a word.
    A.Paraphrase   B.Denotation   C.Central idea   D.Excerpt

75. C   Give an answer; consequence.
    A.Contrast   B.Reproduce   C.Result   D.Key detail

76. C   Words that may not literally mean what they say.
    A.Evidence   B.Cause   C.Figurative language   D.Interpret

77. C   Using few words to give the most important information about something or a complete but brief account of things previously stated.
    A.Attitude   B.Cite   C.Summary   D.Draft

78. A   An explanation for a picture or illustration.
    A.Caption   B.Function   C.Summarize   D.Interpret

79. D   Support; uphold.
    A.Revision   B.Central idea   C.Result   D.Defend

80. D   The reason why something happens.
    A.Plot   B.Function   C.Effect   D.Cause

81. B   Sort; organize.
    A.Event   B.Order   C.Text   D.Hyperbole

82. C   Reason the author writes: persuade, inform, entertain (PIE).
    A.Diagram   B.Italics   C.Authors purpose   D.Result

83. D   Use something to help find a solution.
    A.Develop   B.Claim   C.Diagram   D.Utilize

84. B   To use.
    A.Select   B.Apply   C.Plot   D.Decode

85. A   To make things or ideas known to others; to share or to get ideas across to others.
    A.Convey   B.Detail   C.Claim   D.Evidence

86. B   Explain how things are different.
    A.Complete   B.Contrast   C.Text   D.Claim

87. A   Work out; compute.
    A.Calculate   B.Summary   C.Draft   D.Narrative

88. C   Plain; rough copy.
    A.Infer   B.Result   C.Draft   D.Narrative

89. A To show to be true, to prove.
   A.Establish B.Contrast C.Text structure D.Evidence

90. B A person in a novel, play, or movie or any person, animal or figure represented in a literary work.
   A.Best B.Character C.Outline D.Cause

91. B Give a rough idea; plan.
   A.Evidence B.Outline C.Conclude D.Summarize

92. D The fact of making something seem larger, more important, better, or worse than it really is; overstate the truth.
   A.Paragraph B.Authors purpose C.Order D.Exaggeration

93. C To show or make known.
   A.Function B.Classify C.Reveal D.Calculate

94. A To make a product.
   A.Construct B.Cite C.Explain D.Effective

95. D To find similarities.
   A.Complete B.Sequence C.Categorize D.Compare

96. D To include with something else (e.g. the money is enclosed with the letter in the envelope); to close or hold in.
   A.Calculate B.Best C.Summary D.Enclosed

97. B A simplified drawing.
   A.Reference B.Diagram C.Example D.Draft

98. A To put in a group based on certain characteristics.
   A.Categorize B.Analysis of text C.Response D.Decode

99. B To determine the meaning of.
   A.Examine B.Interpret C.Retell D.Justify

100. A The reading passage.
   A.Text B.Evidence C.Result D.Model

From the words provided for each clue, provide the letter of the word which best matches the clue.

101. C To make a product.
   A.Inference B.Collect C.Create D.Assess

102. D To gather together.
   A.State B.Infer C.Most likely D.Collect

103. A Put in order; arrange.
   A.Organize B.Convince C.Contribute D.Analysis of text

104. B To persuade or get someone to think a certain way.
   A.Support B.Convince C.Narrative D.Imply

105. B What happens because of something.
A.Mood B.Effect C.Suspense D.Result

106. A Name; label.
A.Identify B.Analyze C.Evidence D.Infer

107. B To merge two or more sentences into one sentence.
A.Effect B.Combine sentences C.Paraphrase D.Contrast

108. A The events that make up the story or the main part of the story. The events relate to each other in a pattern or sequence.
A.Plot B.Assess C.Evidence D.Denotation

109. D A comparison of two unlike things using the words "like" or "as".
A.Explain B.Result C.Infer D.Simile

110. B What one thinks about something or somebody.
A.Create B.Opinion C.Establish D.Denotation

111. B To make clear by using examples.
A.Resolution B.Illustrate C.Hyperbole D.Support

112. C To produce words.
A.Discuss B.Infer C.Write D.Connotation

113. D To use a quote from the text to support an idea.
A.Topic B.Describe C.Write D.Cite

114. C Data that uses characteristics.
A.Justify B.Identify C.Quantitative D.Support

115. D What the passage or text is mainly about.
A.Impact B.Narrative C.Perspective D.Central idea

116. D Give good reason; defend.
A.Discuss B.Suspense C.Claim D.Justify

117. A A part of the story that is important.
A.Significance B.State C.Support D.Outline

118. B Reason the author writes: persuade, inform, entertain (PIE).
A.Convey B.Authors purpose C.Organize D.Response

119. C An opinion or the way someone looks at something.
A.Best B.Select C.Perspective D.Qualitative

120. B Exaggeration, not meant to be literal.
A.Interpret B.Hyperbole C.Review D.Distinguish

121. A To make known in detail.
A.Explain B.Define C.Outline D.Examine

122. A Copy; repeat.
A.Reproduce B.Analysis of text C.Calculate D.Text

123. <u>D</u> To choose.
   A.Combine sentences B.Support C.Central idea D.Select

124. <u>A</u> To make a product.
   A.Construct B.Combine sentences C.Key detail D.Most likely

125. <u>C</u> The reason why something happens.
   A.Contrast B.Collect C.Cause D.Caption

126. <u>B</u> Work out; compute.
   A.Observe B.Calculate C.Demonstrate D.Viewpoint

127. <u>A</u> A part of a reading passage.
   A.Excerpt B.Justify C.Figurative language D.Sequence

128. <u>B</u> Sum it up; give a short version.
   A.Qualitative B.Summarize C.Complete D.Convince

129. <u>A</u> The reading passage.
   A.Text B.Support C.Establish D.Review

130. <u>A</u> A way of looking or thinking about something.
   A.Viewpoint B.Hyperbole C.State D.Illustrate

131. <u>A</u> Ending; wrapping up.
   A.Conclusion B.Describe C.Purpose D.Key detail

132. <u>B</u> To provide proof or evidence for.
   A.Purpose B.Support C.Calculate D.Narrative

133. <u>C</u> To put down in writing so that it is saved.
   A.Figurative language B.Text C.Record D.Analyze

134. <u>C</u> Make a good guess; read between the lines.
   A.Key detail B.Illustrate C.Infer D.Review

135. <u>A</u> The ending, answer, or conclusion to a problem or story.
   A.Resolution B.Infer C.Inference D.Interpret

136. <u>D</u> To state a position or declare that something is true or factual, noun-a statement of truth or fact, typically pertaining to an idea that is disputed.
   A.Illustrate B.Narrative C.Explain D.Claim

137. <u>B</u> To show to be true, to prove.
   A.Effect B.Establish C.Calculate D.Construct

138. <u>C</u> A conclusion reached based on reasoning and the use of given facts; a prediction.
   A.Concludes B.Central idea C.Inference D.Valid

139. <u>A</u> A comparison of two unlike things by describing one is the other.
   A.Metaphor B.Explain C.Caption D.Interpret

140. <u>B</u> Give an answer; consequence.
   A.Contrast B.Result C.Sequence D.Construct

141. D   To tell the facts, details.
     A.Contrast B.Support C.Illustrate D.Describe

142. D   Using few words to give the most important information about something or a complete but brief account of things previously stated.
     A.Authors purpose B.Tone C.State D.Summary

143. C   A book or other written work or printed work.
     A.Distinguish B.Effect C.Text D.Suspense

144. D   Look at; study.
     A.Illustrate B.Imply C.Response D.Review

145. C   Give a rough idea; plan.
     A.Describe B.Interpret C.Outline D.Narrative

146. D   A punctuation mark ", " or ',' used at the beginning and ending of text that has been stated from a source.
     A.Describe B.Support C.Examine D.Quotation mark

147. D   Use details from the text to explain your response.
     A.Connotation B.Summary C.Construct D.Support

148. D   Proof; lines and words from text used to prove or disprove an idea.
     A.Denotation B.Demonstrate C.Stanza D.Evidence

149. A   to hint at something without saying it.
     A.Imply B.Demonstrate C.Plot D.Identify

150. C   The subject of discussion or the subject of the article.
     A.Effect B.Convey C.Topic D.Convince

151. C   To look at text carefully by paying attention to its parts, its words, its figurative language, and its tone.
     A.Demonstrate B.Analysis of text C.Analyze D.Resolution

152. D   Tell about; explain.
     A.Convey B.Sequence C.Summarize D.Describe

153. B   To determine the meaning of.
     A.Plot B.Interpret C.Hyperbole D.Tone

154. B   Talk about; argue.
     A.Defend B.Discuss C.Illustrate D.Sequence

155. C   Above all others, most desirable.
     A.Quotation mark B.Simile C.Best D.Discuss

156. B   Look at; inspect.
     A.Summarize B.Examine C.Effect D.Cite

157. D   Describe; characterize.
     A.Collect B.Most likely C.Plot D.Define

158. A   Not sure what is going to happen, waiting.
        A.Suspense   B.Combine sentences   C.Figurative language   D.Contrast

159. D   Words or expression different from literal language, changed or altered to make a
        linguistic point.
        A.Construct   B.Simile   C.Impact   D.Figurative language

160. C   The basic definition or dictionary meaning of a word.
        A.Valid   B.Cite   C.Denotation   D.Write

161. A   Read and examine text in detail looking for important ideas.
        A.Analysis of text   B.Create   C.Most likely   D.Contribute

162. C   A temporary state of mind or feeling.
        A.Central idea   B.Opinion   C.Mood   D.Establish

163. B   Put in order; put in a series.
        A.Cause   B.Sequence   C.Authors purpose   D.Reveal

164. B   Say; affirm.
        A.Claim   B.State   C.Quotation mark   D.Plot

165. A   A restatement of the meaning of a text or passage using other words.
        A.Paraphrase   B.Describe   C.Cite   D.Analysis of text

166. B   To paraphrase or to explain in your own words an important idea or section of text.
        A.Mood   B.Summarize   C.Explain   D.Result

167. C   An explanation for a picture or illustration.
        A.Denotation   B.Distinguish   C.Caption   D.Response

168. D   Support; uphold.
        A.Perspective   B.Interpret   C.Evidence   D.Defend

169. B   Helps to support the central idea in an important way. Authors elaborate using examples or
        anecdotes.
        A.Discuss   B.Key detail   C.Convince   D.Effect

170. A   To cause changes.
        A.Impact   B.Perspective   C.Paraphrase   D.Excerpt

171. C   An answer or reply.
        A.Caption   B.Central idea   C.Response   D.Simile

172. D   A story.
        A.Qualitative   B.Authors purpose   C.Quantitative   D.Narrative

173. C   To make things or ideas known to others; to share or to get ideas across to others.
        A.Mood   B.Perspective   C.Convey   D.Organize

174. A   To show or make known.
        A.Reveal   B.Result   C.Convince   D.Effective

175. B   To consider an idea.
        A.Cite   B.Discuss   C.Establish   D.Convey

176. C All the meanings, associations, emotions, or tones that a word suggests.
A.Distinguish B.Observe C.Connotation D.Narrative

177. B To judge or determine the quality or amount of something.
A.Illustrate B.Evaluate C.Perspective D.Conclusion

178. C Data that is based on numbers.
A.Interpret B.Authors purpose C.Qualitative D.Collect

179. A Sort; organize.
A.Order B.Justify C.Support D.Convey

180. D Proof; information in the text that proves a point.
A.Combine sentences B.Viewpoint C.Central idea D.Evidence

181. B True.
A.Review B.Valid C.Explain D.Discuss

182. D Give the facts; back up with details.
A.Mood B.Describe C.Excerpt D.Support

183. C To find differences.
A.Observe B.Central idea C.Contrast D.Infer

184. B The main point of the story or the text; the unifying element of a story or text, sometimes called main idea or theme.
A.Create B.Central idea C.Reproduce D.Contribute

185. C Judge; consider.
A.Define B.Support C.Assess D.Cite

186. D Will probably happen; probably.
A.Plot B.Combine sentences C.Justify D.Most likely

187. D Able to do its job to the best ability.
A.Best B.Record C.Identify D.Effective

188. A Show; make plain.
A.Demonstrate B.Tone C.Key detail D.Simile

189. B A writer's attitude toward his or her topic which is revealed through specific words used in the text and through figurative language.
A.Support B.Tone C.Concludes D.Paraphrase

190. A To tell or write about something in detail.
A.Describe B.Support C.Quotation mark D.Sequence

191. A To think about carefully and form an opinion.
A.Concludes B.Resolution C.Support D.Infer

192. B To help happen or help cause.
A.Contrast B.Contribute C.Illustrate D.Infer

193. A Finish; end.
A.Complete B.Summarize C.Quotation mark D.Connotation

194. _B_ Make clear; put in your own words.
   A.Central idea B.Explain C.Figurative language D.Inference

195. _C_ A group of lines in a poem (similar to a paragraph).
   A.Opinion B.Infer C.Stanza D.Perspective

196. _D_ To draw or make pictures to explain.
   A.Central idea B.Describe C.Excerpt D.Illustrate

197. _C_ To explain an idea or make a conclusion by looking closely at evidence in text.
   A.Summarize B.Key detail C.Infer D.Discuss

198. _A_ The reason someone does something.
   A.Purpose B.Demonstrate C.Connotation D.Collect

199. _A_ Watch; notice.
   A.Observe B.Examine C.Most likely D.Metaphor

200. _A_ To tell as different.
   A.Distinguish B.Conclusion C.Connotation D.Establish

Matching

Provide the word that best matches each clue.

1. _____ Watch; notice.

2. _____ Describe; characterize.

3. _____ Ending; wrapping up.

4. _____ Think about; wonder about.

5. _____ The reason why something happens.

6. _____ Sum it up; give a short version.

7. _____ To come up with a conclusion without valid evidence to support it.

8. _____ The basic definition or dictionary meaning of a word.

9. _____ To think about carefully and form an opinion.

10. _____ Able to do its job to the best ability.

11. _____ Look at; inspect.

12. _____ Put in order; arrange.

13. _____ The meaning a reader gets from written text.

14. _____ Job, what it does.

15. _____ Give an instance; case.

16. _____ to hint at something without saying it.

17. _____ To make known in detail.

18. _____ Exaggeration, not meant to be literal.

19. _____ Break apart; study the pieces.

20. _____ Read and examine text in detail looking for important ideas.

A. Observe
B. Examine
C. Explain
D. Denotation
E. Conclusion
F. Function
G. Define
H. Reflect
I. Inference
J. Imply
K. Summarize
L. Concludes
M. Hyperbole
N. Effective
O. Organize
P. Analysis of text
Q. Analyze
R. Example
S. Comprehension
T. Cause

Provide the word that best matches each clue.

21. _____ A person who tells something; storyteller.

22. _____ Look at; study.

23. _____ Above all others, most desirable.

24. _____ A form of figurative language and descriptive language that creates a picture in your mind.

25. _____ Repeat; say again.

26. _____ Clearly express something in a speech or writing.

27. _____ Not sure what is going to happen, waiting.

28. _____ All the meanings, associations, emotions, or tones that a word suggests.

29. _____ Put together; create.

30. _____ Data that uses characteristics.

31. _____ Watch; notice.

32. _____ Will probably happen; probably.

33. _____ To explain an idea or make a conclusion by looking closely at evidence in text.

34. _____ Anything that happens, especially something important or unusual.

35. _____ The moment in the story where the conflict reaches its highest point.

36. _____ A part of a reading passage.

37. _____ An answer or reply.

38. _____ To make a product.

39. _____ Make a good guess; read between the lines.

40. _____ To make clear by using examples.

A. Create   B. Infer   C. Image   D. Connotation   E. Most likely
F. Event   G. Best   H. Review   I. Observe   J. Illustrate
K. Formulate   L. Infer   M. Restate   N. Quantitative   O. Suspense
P. Narrator   Q. State   R. Excerpt   S. Climax   T. Response

Provide the word that best matches each clue.

41. _____ A story.

42. _____ To do something the same constantly.

43. _____ Not sure what is going to happen, waiting.

44. _____ Words that may not literally mean what they say.

45. _____ Group; classify.

46. _____ Make out; break apart.

47. _____ Give good reason; defend.

48. _____ To make a product.

49. _____ A group of lines forming the basic unit in a poem; a verse.

50. _____ Sum it up; give a short version.

51. _____ Data that is based on numbers.

52. _____ The subject of discussion or the subject of the article.

53. _____ Imagine; think about.

54. _____ The period and-or location in which a story takes place.

55. _____ To come up with.

56. _____ Reason the author writes: persuade, inform, entertain (PIE).

57. _____ To come up with a conclusion without valid evidence to support it.

58. _____ A single piece of information or fact about something.

59. _____ Judge; consider.

60. _____ Clearly express something in a speech or writing.

A. Consistent	B. Figurative language	C. Detail	D. Inference
E. Decode	F. Authors purpose	G. Evaluate	H. Setting
I. Topic	J. State	K. Sort	L. Visualize
M. Suspense	N. Formulate	O. Justify	P. Narrative
Q. Stanza	R. Qualitative	S. Create	T. Summarize

Provide the word that best matches each clue.

61. _____ Give a rough idea; plan.

62. _____ Read and examine text in detail looking for important ideas.

63. _____ Look at; study.

64. _____ To make a product.

65. _____ The period and-or location in which a story takes place.

66. _____ The ending, answer, or conclusion to a problem or story.

67. _____ To state a position or declare that something is true or factual, noun-a statement of truth or fact, typically pertaining to an idea that is disputed.

68. _____ Describe; characterize.

69. _____ An explanation for a picture or illustration.

70. _____ Repeat; say again.

71. _____ To persuade or get someone to think a certain way.

72. _____ Make out; break apart.

73. _____ To decide.

74. _____ Order in which events, movements, or things follow each other.

75. _____ Watch; notice.

76. _____ A short way of saying what the reading passage is about.

77. _____ Plain; rough copy.

78. _____ A form of figurative language and descriptive language that creates a picture in your mind.

79. _____ Not sure what is going to happen, waiting.

80. _____ A conclusion reached based on reasoning and the use of given facts; a prediction.

A. Analysis of text	B. Suspense	C. Inference	D. Claim
E. Sequence	F. Draft	G. Review	H. Outline
I. Image	J. Define	K. Setting	L. Summary
M. Decode	N. Resolution	O. Restate	P. Convince
Q. Construct	R. Caption	S. Observe	T. Determine

Provide the word that best matches each clue.

81. _____ Look at; inspect.

82. _____ Outline; map out.

83. _____ Tell about; explain.

84. _____ Make a good guess; read between the lines.

85. _____ What the passage or text is mainly about.

86. _____ An answer or reply.

87. _____ A corrected or new version of something written.

88. _____ Break apart; study the pieces.

89. _____ What one thinks about something or somebody.

90. _____ Put in order; sort.

91. _____ to decide based upon information stated in the reading passages.

92. _____ Finish; end.

93. _____ Words that may not literally mean what they say.

94. _____ Explain how things are different.

95. _____ The way a text is presented: introduction, headings and

96. _____ Give an answer; consequence.

97. _____ To produce words.

98. _____ To decide.

99. _____ Put in order; arrange.

100. _____ To help happen or help cause.

A. Trace   B. Examine   C. Describe   D. Text structure
E. Write   F. Conclude   G. Opinion   H. Analyze
I. Determine   J. Response   K. Infer   L. Contrast
M. Result   N. Revision   O. Classify   P. Central idea
Q. Complete   R. Figurative language S. Contribute   T. Organize

Provide the word that best matches each clue.

101. _____ Able to do its job to the best ability.

102. _____ A restatement of the meaning of a text or passage using other words.

103. _____ Think about; wonder about.

104. _____ The main point of the story or the text; the unifying element of a story or text, sometimes called main idea or theme.

105. _____ Make out; break apart.

106. _____ A word, phrase or clause used to describe or qualify another word, phrase or clause.

107. _____ To show or make known.

108. _____ What happens because of something.

109. _____ Sort; organize.

110. _____ To cause changes.

111. _____ Describe; characterize.

112. _____ To find differences.

113. _____ An opinion or the way someone looks at something.

114. _____ to hint at something without saying it.

115. _____ Group; classify.

116. _____ Make a good guess; read between the lines.

117. _____ Give the facts; back up with details.

118. _____ A punctuation mark ", " or ',' used at the beginning and ending of text that has been stated from a source.

119. _____ A person in a novel, play, or movie or any person, animal or figure represented in a literary work.

120. _____ An explanation for a picture or illustration.

A. Support	B. Quotation mark	C. Reflect	D. Caption
E. Sort	F. Perspective	G. Decode	H. Modifier
I. Effective	J. Effect	K. Infer	L. Order
M. Contrast	N. Reveal	O. Define	P. Character
Q. Paraphrase	R. Imply	S. Impact	T. Central idea

Provide the word that best matches each clue.

121. _____ To state a position or declare that something is true or factual, noun-a statement of truth or fact, typically pertaining to an idea that is disputed.

122. _____ A simplified drawing.

123. _____ To determine and mark points on a graph.

124. _____ The basic definition or dictionary meaning of a word.

125. _____ A comparison of two unlike things using the words "like" or "as".

126. _____ Words that may not literally mean what they say.

127. _____ A part of a reading passage.

128. _____ To paraphrase or to explain in your own words an important idea or section of text.

129. _____ The reason why something happens.

130. _____ To prove.

131. _____ The ending, answer, or conclusion to a problem or story.

132. _____ Group; classify.

133. _____ A person who tells something; storyteller.

134. _____ Copy; repeat.

135. _____ To come up with a conclusion without valid evidence to support it.

136. _____ Plain; rough copy.

137. _____ The moment in the story where the conflict reaches its highest point.

138. _____ Sum it up; give a short version.

139. _____ The events that make up the story or the main part of the story. The events relate to each other in a pattern or sequence.

140. _____ The subject of discussion or the subject of the article.

A. Summarize	B. Denotation	C. Excerpt	D. Cause
E. Reproduce	F. Sort	G. Plot	H. Topic
I. Narrator	J. Climax	K. Justify	L. Draft
M. Figurative language	N. Plot	O. Inference	P. Summarize
Q. Diagram	R. Resolution	S. Simile	T. Claim

Provide the word that best matches each clue.

141. _____ To show or make known.

142. _____ Think about; wonder about.

143. _____ Tell how alike; judge against.

144. _____ Reason the author writes: persuade, inform, entertain (PIE).

145. _____ A usually short piece of written work that focuses on a topic.

146. _____ Repeat; say again.

147. _____ The reading passage.

148. _____ Repeat; say again.

149. _____ To change something to work in a certain way.

150. _____ Record; name.

151. _____ Change; alter.

152. _____ A group of lines forming the basic unit in a poem; a verse.

153. _____ Put together; create.

154. _____ To explain an idea or make a conclusion by looking closely at evidence in text.

155. _____ Give good reason; defend.

156. _____ Look at; inspect.

157. _____ Support; uphold.

158. _____ A group of words within a text.

159. _____ Data that is based on numbers.

160. _____ To find similarities.

A. Stanza	B. Text	C. Infer	D. Restate
E. Qualitative	F. Authors purpose	G. Manipulate	H. Defend
I. Phrase	J. Examine	K. List	L. Compare
M. Reflect	N. Justify	O. Formulate	P. Reveal
Q. Passage	R. Compare	S. Retell	T. Revise

Provide the word that best matches each clue.

161. _____ To help happen or help cause.

162. _____ An explanation for a picture or illustration.

163. _____ The period and-or location in which a story takes place.

164. _____ Put in order; sort.

165. _____ Exaggeration, not meant to be literal.

166. _____ Proof; lines and words from text used to prove or disprove an idea.

167. _____ A section of writing consisting of one or more sentences grouped together and discussing one main subject.

168. _____ What one thinks about something or somebody.

169. _____ To decide.

170. _____ Exact or specific.

171. _____ A person in a novel, play, or movie or any person, animal or figure represented in a literary work.

172. _____ Will probably happen; probably.

173. _____ The moment in the story where the conflict reaches its highest point.

174. _____ Words or expression different from literal language, changed or altered to make a linguistic point.

175. _____ Give an instance; case.

176. _____ A usually short piece of written work that focuses on a topic.

177. _____ Clearly express something in a speech or writing.

178. _____ To do something the same constantly.

179. _____ To make known in detail.

180. _____ Group; classify.

A. Character	B. Precise	C. Contribute	D. Consistent
E. Evidence	F. Figurative language	G. Caption	H. Setting
I. Example	J. State	K. Most likely	L. Sort
M. Explain	N. Passage	O. Paragraph	P. Opinion
Q. Classify	R. Climax	S. Hyperbole	T. Determine

Provide the word that best matches each clue.

181. _____ Words or expression different from literal language, changed or altered to make a linguistic point.

182. _____ Using few words to give the most important information about something or a complete but brief account of things previously stated.

183. _____ A book, person, or document used to provide information or data.

184. _____ Able to do its job to the best ability.

185. _____ Put in order; arrange.

186. _____ Proof; lines and words from text used to prove or disprove an idea.

187. _____ The subject of discussion or the subject of the article.

188. _____ Exaggeration, not meant to be literal.

189. _____ Describe; characterize.

190. _____ To make clear by using examples.

191. _____ Name; label.

192. _____ To determine and mark points on a graph.

193. _____ To connect back to another text.

194. _____ What happens because of something.

195. _____ A group of lines forming the basic unit in a poem; a verse.

196. _____ Look at; inspect.

197. _____ Work out; compute.

198. _____ To explain an idea or make a conclusion by looking closely at evidence in text.

199. _____ To come up with a conclusion without valid evidence to support it.

200. _____ Words that may not literally mean what they say.

A. Topic	B. Source	C. Plot	D. Calculate
E. Reference	F. Figurative language	G. Organize	H. Summary
I. Examine	J. Hyperbole	K. Effective	L. Effect
M. Identify	N. Evidence	O. Inference	P. Illustrate
Q. Stanza	R. Define	S. Figurative language	T. Infer

Provide the word that best matches each clue.

1. OBSERVE   Watch; notice.

2. DEFINE   Describe; characterize.

3. CONCLUSION   Ending; wrapping up.

4. REFLECT   Think about; wonder about.

5. CAUSE   The reason why something happens.

6. SUMMARIZE   Sum it up; give a short version.

7. INFERENCE   To come up with a conclusion without valid evidence to support it.

8. DENOTATION   The basic definition or dictionary meaning of a word.

9. CONCLUDES   To think about carefully and form an opinion.

10. EFFECTIVE   Able to do its job to the best ability.

11. EXAMINE   Look at; inspect.

12. ORGANIZE   Put in order; arrange.

13. COMPREHENSION   The meaning a reader gets from written text.

14. FUNCTION   Job, what it does.

15. EXAMPLE   Give an instance; case.

16. IMPLY   to hint at something without saying it.

17. EXPLAIN   To make known in detail.

18. HYPERBOLE   Exaggeration, not meant to be literal.

19. ANALYZE   Break apart; study the pieces.

20. ANALYSIS OF TEXT   Read and examine text in detail looking for important ideas.

A. Observe	B. Examine	C. Explain	D. Denotation
E. Conclusion	F. Function	G. Define	H. Reflect
I. Inference	J. Imply	K. Summarize	L. Concludes
M. Hyperbole	N. Effective	O. Organize	P. Analysis of text
Q. Analyze	R. Example	S. Comprehension	T. Cause

Provide the word that best matches each clue.

21. NARRATOR   A person who tells something; storyteller.

22. REVIEW   Look at; study.

23. BEST   Above all others, most desirable.

24. IMAGE _____ A form of figurative language and descriptive language that creates a picture in your mind.

25. RESTATE _____ Repeat; say again.

26. STATE _____ Clearly express something in a speech or writing.

27. SUSPENSE _____ Not sure what is going to happen, waiting.

28. CONNOTATION _____ All the meanings, associations, emotions, or tones that a word suggests.

29. FORMULATE _____ Put together; create.

30. QUANTITATIVE _____ Data that uses characteristics.

31. OBSERVE _____ Watch; notice.

32. MOST LIKELY _____ Will probably happen; probably.

33. INFER _____ To explain an idea or make a conclusion by looking closely at evidence in text.

34. EVENT _____ Anything that happens, especially something important or unusual.

35. CLIMAX _____ The moment in the story where the conflict reaches its highest point.

36. EXCERPT _____ A part of a reading passage.

37. RESPONSE _____ An answer or reply.

38. CREATE _____ To make a product.

39. INFER _____ Make a good guess; read between the lines.

40. ILLUSTRATE _____ To make clear by using examples.

A. Create	B. Infer	C. Image	D. Connotation	E. Most likely
F. Event	G. Best	H. Review	I. Observe	J. Illustrate
K. Formulate	L. Infer	M. Restate	N. Quantitative	O. Suspense
P. Narrator	Q. State	R. Excerpt	S. Climax	T. Response

Provide the word that best matches each clue.

41. NARRATIVE _____ A story.

42. CONSISTENT _____ To do something the same constantly.

43. SUSPENSE _____ Not sure what is going to happen, waiting.

44. FIGURATIVE LANGUAGE Words that may not literally mean what they say.

45. SORT _____ Group; classify.

46. DECODE _____ Make out; break apart.

47. JUSTIFY _____ Give good reason; defend.

48. CREATE _____ To make a product.

49. STANZA _____ A group of lines forming the basic unit in a poem; a verse.

50. SUMMARIZE _____ Sum it up; give a short version.

51. QUALITATIVE _____ Data that is based on numbers.

52. TOPIC _____ The subject of discussion or the subject of the article.

53. VISUALIZE _____ Imagine; think about.

54. SETTING _____ The period and-or location in which a story takes place.

55. FORMULATE _____ To come up with.

56. AUTHORS PURPOSE _____ Reason the author writes: persuade, inform, entertain (PIE).

57. INFERENCE _____ To come up with a conclusion without valid evidence to support it.

58. DETAIL _____ A single piece of information or fact about something.

59. EVALUATE _____ Judge; consider.

60. STATE _____ Clearly express something in a speech or writing.

A. Consistent	B. Figurative language	C. Detail	D. Inference
E. Decode	F. Authors purpose	G. Evaluate	H. Setting
I. Topic	J. State	K. Sort	L. Visualize
M. Suspense	N. Formulate	O. Justify	P. Narrative
Q. Stanza	R. Qualitative	S. Create	T. Summarize

Provide the word that best matches each clue.

61. OUTLINE _____ Give a rough idea; plan.

62. ANALYSIS OF TEXT _____ Read and examine text in detail looking for important ideas.

63. REVIEW _____ Look at; study.

64. CONSTRUCT _____ To make a product.

65. SETTING _____ The period and-or location in which a story takes place.

66. RESOLUTION _____ The ending, answer, or conclusion to a problem or story.

67. CLAIM _____ To state a position or declare that something is true or factual, noun-a statement of truth or fact, typically pertaining to an idea that is disputed.

68. DEFINE _____ Describe; characterize.

69. CAPTION _____ An explanation for a picture or illustration.

70. RESTATE _____ Repeat; say again.

71. CONVINCE _____ To persuade or get someone to think a certain way.

72. DECODE _____ Make out; break apart.

73. DETERMINE _____ To decide.

74. SEQUENCE _____ Order in which events, movements, or things follow each other.

75. OBSERVE _____ Watch; notice.

76. SUMMARY _____ A short way of saying what the reading passage is about.

77. DRAFT _____ Plain; rough copy.

78. IMAGE _____ A form of figurative language and descriptive language that creates a picture in your mind.

79. SUSPENSE _____ Not sure what is going to happen, waiting.

80. INFERENCE _____ A conclusion reached based on reasoning and the use of given facts; a prediction.

A. Analysis of text   B. Suspense   C. Inference   D. Claim
E. Sequence   F. Draft   G. Review   H. Outline
I. Image   J. Define   K. Setting   L. Summary
M. Decode   N. Resolution   O. Restate   P. Convince
Q. Construct   R. Caption   S. Observe   T. Determine

Provide the word that best matches each clue.

81. EXAMINE _____ Look at; inspect.

82. TRACE _____ Outline; map out.

83. DESCRIBE _____ Tell about; explain.

84. INFER _____ Make a good guess; read between the lines.

85. CENTRAL IDEA _____ What the passage or text is mainly about.

86. RESPONSE _____ An answer or reply.

87. REVISION _____ A corrected or new version of something written.

88. ANALYZE _____ Break apart; study the pieces.

89. OPINION _____ What one thinks about something or somebody.

90. CLASSIFY _____ Put in order; sort.

91. CONCLUDE _____ to decide based upon information stated in the reading passages.

92. COMPLETE _____ Finish; end.

93. FIGURATIVE LANGUAGE Words that may not literally mean what they say.

94. CONTRAST _____ Explain how things are different.

95. TEXT STRUCTURE _____ The way a text is presented: introduction, headings and

96. RESULT _____ Give an answer; consequence.

97. WRITE _____ To produce words.

98. DETERMINE _____ To decide.

99. ORGANIZE _____ Put in order; arrange.

100. CONTRIBUTE _____ To help happen or help cause.

A. Trace	B. Examine	C. Describe	D. Text structure
E. Write	F. Conclude	G. Opinion	H. Analyze
I. Determine	J. Response	K. Infer	L. Contrast
M. Result	N. Revision	O. Classify	P. Central idea
Q. Complete	R. Figurative language	S. Contribute	T. Organize

Provide the word that best matches each clue.

101. EFFECTIVE _____ Able to do its job to the best ability.

102. PARAPHRASE _____ A restatement of the meaning of a text or passage using other words.

103. REFLECT _____ Think about; wonder about.

104. CENTRAL IDEA _____ The main point of the story or the text; the unifying element of a story or text, sometimes called main idea or theme.

105. DECODE _____ Make out; break apart.

106. MODIFIER _____ A word, phrase or clause used to describe or qualify another word, phrase or clause.

107. REVEAL _____ To show or make known.

108. EFFECT _____ What happens because of something.

109. ORDER _____ Sort; organize.

110. IMPACT _____ To cause changes.

111. DEFINE _____ Describe; characterize.

112. CONTRAST _____ To find differences.

113. PERSPECTIVE _____ An opinion or the way someone looks at something.

114. IMPLY _____ to hint at something without saying it.

115. SORT _____ Group; classify.

116. INFER _____ Make a good guess; read between the lines.

117. SUPPORT _____ Give the facts; back up with details.

118. QUOTATION MARK _____ A punctuation mark ", " or ',' used at the beginning and ending of text that has been stated from a source.

119. CHARACTER _____ A person in a novel, play, or movie or any person, animal or figure represented in a literary work.

120. CAPTION _____ An explanation for a picture or illustration.

A. Support	B. Quotation mark	C. Reflect	D. Caption
E. Sort	F. Perspective	G. Decode	H. Modifier
I. Effective	J. Effect	K. Infer	L. Order
M. Contrast	N. Reveal	O. Define	P. Character
Q. Paraphrase	R. Imply	S. Impact	T. Central idea

Provide the word that best matches each clue.

121. CLAIM _____ To state a position or declare that something is true or factual, noun-a statement of truth or fact, typically pertaining to an idea that is disputed.

122. DIAGRAM _____ A simplified drawing.

123. PLOT _____ To determine and mark points on a graph.

124. DENOTATION _____ The basic definition or dictionary meaning of a word.

125. SIMILE _____ A comparison of two unlike things using the words "like" or "as".

126. FIGURATIVE LANGUAGE _____ Words that may not literally mean what they say.

127. EXCERPT _____ A part of a reading passage.

128. SUMMARIZE _____ To paraphrase or to explain in your own words an important idea or section of text.

129. CAUSE _____ The reason why something happens.

130. JUSTIFY _____ To prove.

131. RESOLUTION _____ The ending, answer, or conclusion to a problem or story.

132. SORT _____ Group; classify.

133. NARRATOR _____ A person who tells something; storyteller.

134. REPRODUCE _____ Copy; repeat.

135. INFERENCE _____ To come up with a conclusion without valid evidence to support it.

136. DRAFT _____ Plain; rough copy.

137. CLIMAX _____ The moment in the story where the conflict reaches its highest point.

138. SUMMARIZE _____ Sum it up; give a short version.

139. PLOT _____ The events that make up the story or the main part of the story. The events relate to each other in a pattern or sequence.

140. TOPIC _____ The subject of discussion or the subject of the article.

A. Summarize	B. Denotation	C. Excerpt	D. Cause
E. Reproduce	F. Sort	G. Plot	H. Topic
I. Narrator	J. Climax	K. Justify	L. Draft
M. Figurative language	N. Plot	O. Inference	P. Summarize
Q. Diagram	R. Resolution	S. Simile	T. Claim

Provide the word that best matches each clue.

141. REVEAL _____ To show or make known.

142. REFLECT _____ Think about; wonder about.

143. COMPARE _____ Tell how alike; judge against.

144. AUTHORS PURPOSE _____ Reason the author writes: persuade, inform, entertain (PIE).

145. PASSAGE _____ A usually short piece of written work that focuses on a topic.

146. RESTATE _____ Repeat; say again.

147. TEXT _____ The reading passage.

148. RETELL _____ Repeat; say again.

149. MANIPULATE _____ To change something to work in a certain way.

150. LIST _____ Record; name.

151. REVISE _____ Change; alter.

152. STANZA _____ A group of lines forming the basic unit in a poem; a verse.

153. FORMULATE _____ Put together; create.

154. INFER _____ To explain an idea or make a conclusion by looking closely at evidence in text.

155. JUSTIFY _____ Give good reason; defend.

156. EXAMINE _____ Look at; inspect.

157. DEFEND _____ Support; uphold.

158. PHRASE _____ A group of words within a text.

159. QUALITATIVE _____ Data that is based on numbers.

160. COMPARE _____ To find similarities.

A. Stanza	B. Text	C. Infer	D. Restate
E. Qualitative	F. Authors purpose	G. Manipulate	H. Defend
I. Phrase	J. Examine	K. List	L. Compare
M. Reflect	N. Justify	O. Formulate	P. Reveal
Q. Passage	R. Compare	S. Retell	T. Revise

Provide the word that best matches each clue.

161. CONTRIBUTE _____ To help happen or help cause.

162. CAPTION _____ An explanation for a picture or illustration.

163. SETTING _____ The period and-or location in which a story takes place.

164. CLASSIFY _____ Put in order; sort.

165. HYPERBOLE _____ Exaggeration, not meant to be literal.

166. EVIDENCE _____ Proof; lines and words from text used to prove or disprove an idea.

167. PARAGRAPH _____ A section of writing consisting of one or more sentences grouped together and discussing one main subject.

168. OPINION _____ What one thinks about something or somebody.

169. DETERMINE _____ To decide.

170. PRECISE _____ Exact or specific.

171. CHARACTER _____ A person in a novel, play, or movie or any person, animal or figure represented in a literary work.

172. MOST LIKELY _____ Will probably happen; probably.

173. CLIMAX _____ The moment in the story where the conflict reaches its highest point.

174. FIGURATIVE LANGUAGE _____ Words or expression different from literal language, changed or altered to make a linguistic point.

175. EXAMPLE _____ Give an instance; case.

176. PASSAGE _____ A usually short piece of written work that focuses on a topic.

177. STATE _____ Clearly express something in a speech or writing.

178. CONSISTENT _____ To do something the same constantly.

179. EXPLAIN _____ To make known in detail.

180. SORT _____ Group; classify.

A. Character	B. Precise	C. Contribute	D. Consistent
E. Evidence	F. Figurative language	G. Caption	H. Setting
I. Example	J. State	K. Most likely	L. Sort
M. Explain	N. Passage	O. Paragraph	P. Opinion
Q. Classify	R. Climax	S. Hyperbole	T. Determine

Provide the word that best matches each clue.

181. FIGURATIVE LANGUAGE _____ Words or expression different from literal language, changed or altered to make a linguistic point.

182. SUMMARY _____ Using few words to give the most important information about something or a complete but brief account of things previously stated.

183. SOURCE _____ A book, person, or document used to provide information or data.

184. EFFECTIVE _____ Able to do its job to the best ability.

185. ORGANIZE _____ Put in order; arrange.

186. EVIDENCE _____ Proof; lines and words from text used to prove or disprove an idea.

187. TOPIC _____ The subject of discussion or the subject of the article.

188. HYPERBOLE _____ Exaggeration, not meant to be literal.

189. DEFINE _____ Describe; characterize.

190. ILLUSTRATE _____ To make clear by using examples.

191. IDENTIFY _____ Name; label.

192. PLOT _____ To determine and mark points on a graph.

193. REFERENCE _____ To connect back to another text.

194. EFFECT _____ What happens because of something.

195. STANZA _____ A group of lines forming the basic unit in a poem; a verse.

196. EXAMINE _____ Look at; inspect.

197. CALCULATE _____ Work out; compute.

198. INFER _____ To explain an idea or make a conclusion by looking closely at evidence in text.

199. INFERENCE _____ To come up with a conclusion without valid evidence to support it.

200. FIGURATIVE LANGUAGE _____ Words that may not literally mean what they say.

A. Topic
B. Source
C. Plot
D. Calculate
E. Reference
F. Figurative language
G. Organize
H. Summary
I. Examine
J. Hyperbole
K. Effective
L. Effect
M. Identify
N. Evidence
O. Inference
P. Illustrate
Q. Stanza
R. Define
S. Figurative language
T. Infer

Word Search

1. *Find the hidden words. The words have been placed horizontally, vertically, or diagonally. When you locate a word, draw a circle around it.*

R	S	F	O	R	M	U	L	A	T	E	R	E	C	O	G	N	I	Z	E
C	E	D	E	S	C	R	I	B	E	V	V	N	I	N	V	A	L	I	D
K	X	O	H	Y	P	E	R	B	O	L	E	R	T	X	H	E	R	C	X
X	C	O	M	P	L	E	T	E	A	O	M	Z	O	N	H	O	V	X	F
C	O	M	P	A	R	E	E	T	S	V	C	W	N	I	L	A	K	H	U
O	D	E	S	C	R	I	B	E	S	P	R	N	E	R	Y	Y	E	H	N
L	R	E	L	I	A	B	L	E	E	B	C	L	I	M	A	X	M	X	C
T	P	V	X	F	I	E	D	L	S	I	N	T	E	R	P	R	E	T	T
O	L	J	Y	R	U	O	U	R	S	I	N	F	E	R	E	N	C	E	I
I	O	L	H	T	J	O	H	G	A	V	B	P	C	G	J	V	R	W	O
C	T	H	C	L	A	S	S	I	F	Y	Z	J	U	S	T	I	F	Y	N
C	O	N	T	R	A	S	T	S	U	P	P	O	R	T	D	D	W	H	V

1. A writer's attitude toward his or her topic which is revealed through specific words used in the text and through figurative language.
2. Judge; consider.
3. The moment in the story where the conflict reaches its highest point.
4. Give the facts; back up with details.
5. Tell how things are different; draw a distinction.
6. Finish; end.
7. Give good reason; defend.
8. To determine the meaning of.
9. Able to trust.
10. To come up with.
11. To identify from knowledge of appearance or characteristics.
12. Not true.
13. arrange (a group of people or things) in classes or categories according to shared qualities or characteristics.
14. Job, what it does.
15. The events that make up the story or the main part of the story. The events relate to each other in a pattern or sequence.
16. Tell how alike; judge against.
17. To come up with a conclusion without valid evidence to support it.
18. To tell or write about something in detail.
19. Exaggeration, not meant to be literal.
20. Tell about; explain.

A. Contrast	B. Assess	C. Climax	D. Plot	E. Interpret	F. Tone	G. Recognize
H. Invalid	I. Inference	J. Justify	K. Formulate	L. Reliable	M. Hyperbole	N. Describe
O. Complete	P. Classify	Q. Compare	R. Support	S. Function	T. Describe	

2. *Find the hidden words. The words have been placed horizontally, vertically, or diagonally. When you locate a word, draw a circle around it.*

Z	F	T	C	O	M	B	I	N	E	S	E	N	T	E	N	C	E	S	W
G	X	J	C	D	N	P	A	S	S	A	G	E	Y	Z	U	T	S	T	N
E	E	O	O	S	U	M	M	A	R	Y	R	E	N	C	N	O	T	J	H
N	A	D	N	Z	E	Y	S	M	D	E	F	E	N	D	N	N	A	R	F
E	D	I	S	L	V	P	T	S	I	N	V	A	L	I	D	E	N	P	M
R	I	N	I	O	A	R	A	E	C	M	E	X	R	M	O	I	Z	R	J
A	S	A	S	Y	L	E	T	Q	I	Y	S	I	Y	Q	T	T	A	E	M
L	C	R	T	F	U	D	E	U	Q	W	Y	X	P	V	S	R	J	C	G
I	U	A	E	P	A	I	M	E	E	A	P	A	S	S	E	S	S	I	K
Z	S	A	N	U	T	C	Z	N	Q	M	E	T	A	P	H	O	R	S	C
E	S	B	T	P	E	T	N	C	V	J	C	O	N	C	L	U	D	E	S
G	C	O	M	P	L	E	T	E	R	S	K	E	Y	D	E	T	A	I	L

1. Guess; tell what will happen next.
2. A writer's attitude toward his or her topic which is revealed through specific words used in the text and through figurative language.
3. A short way of saying what the reading passage is about.
4. A comparison of two unlike things by describing one is the other.
5. Say; affirm.
6. to make a statement based upon details from the reading passage that might be true in other situations.
7. Support; uphold.
8. A usually short piece of written work that focuses on a topic.
9. To judge or determine the quality or amount of something.
10. A group of lines forming the basic unit in a poem; a verse.
11. Helps to support the central idea in an important way. Authors elaborate using examples or anecdotes.
12. Finish; end.
13. To consider an idea.
14. To merge two or more sentences into one sentence.
15. To do something the same constantly.
16. Judge; consider.
17. Order in which events, movements, or things follow each other.
18. Exact or specific.
19. To think about carefully and form an opinion.
20. Not true.

A. Stanza
F. Discuss
K. Defend
P. Passage

B. Sequence
G. Tone
L. State
Q. Generalize

C. Metaphor
H. Invalid
M. Assess
R. Summary

D. Evaluate
I. Combine sentences
N. Predict
S. Key detail

E. Complete
J. Concludes
O. Consistent
T. Precise

3. *Find the hidden words. The words have been placed horizontally, vertically, or diagonally. When you locate a word, draw a circle around it.*

S	A	R	I	T	A	L	I	C	S	I	L	L	U	S	T	R	A	T	E
S	X	E	F	O	R	M	U	L	A	T	E	W	W	H	Y	U	X	T	Q
U	R	F	R	D	E	S	C	R	I	B	E	S	E	X	A	M	I	N	E
M	I	L	I	E	G	E	Y	B	I	S	S	E	V	I	D	E	N	C	E
M	S	E	S	S	O	N	V	J	M	T	J	U	L	M	Z	R	N	D	Z
A	S	C	P	T	H	S	Q	Q	O	A	D	I	S	C	U	S	S	E	O
R	R	T	D	A	B	J	Y	K	D	N	J	H	F	O	E	H	Q	V	P
I	E	J	A	B	I	E	I	I	E	Z	R	E	L	I	A	B	L	E	I
Z	C	M	P	L	K	C	H	D	L	A	S	O	R	T	S	A	E	L	N
E	O	I	Q	I	R	C	E	N	T	R	A	L	I	D	E	A	W	O	I
G	R	K	R	S	P	P	E	R	S	P	E	C	T	I	V	E	Q	P	O
J	D	P	D	H	R	E	S	O	L	U	T	I	O	N	M	B	D	F	N

1. Group; classify.
2. A group of lines forming the basic unit in a poem; a verse.
3. To show to be true, to prove.
4. Talk about; argue.
5. To tell or write about something in detail.
6. Proof; lines and words from text used to prove or disprove an idea.
7. To put down in writing so that it is saved.
8. The ending, answer, or conclusion to a problem or story.
9. What the passage or text is mainly about.
10. To draw or make pictures to explain.
11. Put together; create.
12. To paraphrase or to explain in your own words an important idea or section of text.
13. Think about; wonder about.
14. Look at; inspect.
15. An opinion or the way someone looks at something.
16. A style of print where the letters slope to the right; may be used to emphasize or to indicate the title of published work.
17. What one thinks about something or somebody.
18. To work out, grow, or expand.
19. To represent something that will serve as an example.
20. Able to trust.

A. Reflect
B. Opinion
C. Establish
D. Record
E. Illustrate
F. Describe
G. Central idea
H. Sort
I. Resolution
J. Italics
K. Summarize
L. Perspective
M. Model
N. Evidence
O. Reliable
P. Stanza
Q. Develop
R. Discuss
S. Formulate
T. Examine

4. *Find the hidden words. The words have been placed horizontally, vertically, or diagonally. When you locate a word, draw a circle around it.*

G	E	I	H	N	Q	S	U	P	P	O	R	T	A	S	S	E	S	S	N
C	G	Y	F	A	M	O	S	T	L	I	K	E	L	Y	F	J	A	T	F
A	G	K	E	E	Y	M	P	E	X	I	S	C	I	T	E	U	B	F	S
T	E	C	L	S	C	A	R	F	V	S	E	F	A	O	G	S	X	A	Z
E	V	O	J	T	O	N	S	F	R	S	Q	C	K	X	A	T	K	M	O
G	I	N	X	A	N	I	E	E	S	J	U	C	A	P	T	I	O	N	S
O	D	S	H	B	C	P	C	T	O	E	I	Y	D	C	F	P	C	Y	
R	E	T	S	L	L	U	O	T	A	I	N	F	E	R	T	Y	F	M	Y
I	N	R	D	I	U	L	T	I	N	G	C	C	L	A	S	S	I	F	Y
Z	C	U	X	S	D	A	R	V	Z	N	E	G	R	E	C	O	R	D	N
E	E	C	M	H	E	T	K	E	A	N	A	R	R	A	T	O	R	A	V
F	W	T	U	Q	S	E	J	M	S	C	L	A	S	S	I	F	Y	L	S

1. Will probably happen; probably.
2. A group of lines forming the basic unit in a poem; a verse.
3. To prove.
4. Able to do its job to the best ability.
5. To think about carefully and form an opinion.
6. Place in a class or group.
7. An explanation for a picture or illustration.
8. To show to be true, to prove.
9. Put in order; sort.
10. arrange (a group of people or things) in classes or categories according to shared qualities or characteristics.
11. Proof; lines and words from text used to prove or disprove an idea.
12. To use a quote from the text to support an idea.
13. A person who tells something; storyteller.
14. To put down in writing so that it is saved.
15. To change something to work in a certain way.
16. Make a good guess; read between the lines.
17. Judge; consider.
18. Order in which events, movements, or things follow each other.
19. To make a product.
20. To provide proof or evidence for.

A. Support   B. Construct   C. Effective   D. Sequence   E. Infer   F. Establish   G. Concludes
H. Caption   I. Evidence   J. Record   K. Justify   L. Assess   M. Narrator   N. Most likely
O. Cite   P. Manipulate   Q. Stanza   R. Categorize   S. Classify   T. Classify

5. *Find the hidden words. The words have been placed horizontally, vertically, or diagonally. When you locate a word, draw a circle around it.*

O	B	V	G	R	D	P	U	S	C	O	N	C	L	U	S	I	O	N	J
W	E	U	Y	E	N	K	E	U	X	M	B	U	W	B	W	O	C	H	A
I	R	J	F	V	D	B	E	M	G	M	B	S	T	A	T	E	G	P	S
L	E	R	M	I	K	Q	O	M	I	N	F	E	R	E	N	C	E	X	S
L	L	L	O	S	D	Q	F	A	G	V	I	S	U	A	L	I	Z	E	E
U	I	X	D	E	S	L	Q	R	S	D	E	S	C	R	I	B	E	X	S
S	A	D	E	C	O	D	E	I	L	Y	O	R	S	C	A	U	S	E	S
T	B	N	L	T	Y	T	K	Z	D	E	S	C	R	I	B	E	Q	H	R
R	L	S	O	U	R	C	E	C	O	N	N	O	T	A	T	I	O	N	
A	E	F	I	G	U	R	A	T	I	V	E	L	A	N	G	U	A	G	E
T	Y	R	E	C	O	R	D	H	C	E	N	T	R	A	L	I	D	E	A
E	X	G	V	M	A	U	T	H	O	R	S	P	U	R	P	O	S	E	N

1. Change; alter.
2. To make clear by using examples.
3. Sum it up; give a short version.
4. To tell or write about something in detail.
5. Ending; wrapping up.
6. Judge; consider.
7. The reason why something happens.
8. Reason the author writes: persuade, inform, entertain (PIE).
9. Imagine; think about.
10. Make out; break apart.
11. To tell the facts, details.
12. To represent something that will serve as an example.
13. A conclusion reached based on reasoning and the use of given facts; a prediction.
14. Say; affirm.
15. Able to trust.
16. All the meanings, associations, emotions, or tones that a word suggests.
17. A book, person, or document used to provide information or data.
18. Words that may not literally mean what they say.
19. To put down in writing so that it is saved.
20. What the passage or text is mainly about.

A. Authors purpose
E. Source
I. State
M. Figurative language
Q. Visualize

B. Illustrate
F. Reliable
J. Assess
N. Record
R. Describe

C. Central idea
G. Describe
K. Conclusion
O. Inference
S. Decode

D. Connotation
H. Model
L. Cause
P. Summarize
T. Revise

6. *Find the hidden words. The words have been placed horizontally, vertically, or diagonally. When you locate a word, draw a circle around it.*

S	S	S	M	O	D	I	F	I	E	R	V	M	W	L	X	F	I	E	W
O	E	U	K	Q	T	N	I	G	R	E	T	E	L	L	U	O	M	X	O
U	Q	P	R	R	W	J	E	R	R	U	O	U	T	L	I	N	E	A	R
R	U	P	E	E	N	U	V	S	E	Q	U	E	N	C	E	W	Y	G	E
C	E	O	V	S	D	S	G	R	Y	Z	L	C	P	D	F	B	A	G	F
E	N	R	I	U	E	T	T	E	X	T	Z	O	S	D	B	D	T	E	E
U	C	T	S	L	S	I	M	L	E	W	O	N	T	E	T	D	T	R	R
Q	E	D	I	T	C	F	Y	I	K	E	T	V	A	F	O	K	I	A	E
S	Y	I	O	W	R	Y	E	A	S	I	P	E	T	I	P	A	T	T	N
H	C	Y	N	K	I	E	D	B	J	D	E	Y	E	N	I	V	U	I	C
M	J	U	K	Z	B	U	C	L	R	X	R	X	N	E	C	C	D	O	E
F	P	T	R	U	E	J	X	E	G	T	N	T	F	C	Y	D	E	N	Y

1. To prove.
2. Put in order; put in a series.
3. The subject of discussion or the subject of the article.
4. Give an answer; consequence.
5. Give the facts; back up with details.
6. Describe; characterize.
7. A book, person, or document used to provide information or data.
8. To connect back to another text.
9. The reading passage.
10. To make things or ideas known to others; to share or to get ideas across to others.
11. Able to trust.
12. Give a rough idea; plan.
13. A word, phrase or clause used to describe or qualify another word, phrase or clause.
14. Order in which events, movements, or things follow each other.
15. The fact of making something seem larger, more important, better, or worse than it really is; overstate the truth.
16. Tell about; explain.
17. Repeat; say again.
18. A corrected or new version of something written.
19. Clearly express something in a speech or writing.
20. The way someone feels about something.

A. Attitude   B. Justify   C. Exaggeration   D. Support   E. Revision   F. Convey
G. Sequence   H. Define   I. Reliable   J. Outline   K. Source   L. Modifier
M. Retell   N. Result   O. Text   P. State   Q. Describe   R. Sequence
S. Topic   T. Reference

7. *Find the hidden words. The words have been placed horizontally, vertically, or diagonally. When you locate a word, draw a circle around it.*

E	X	P	L	I	C	I	T	M	U	O	V	G	J	G	B	X	O	P	J
I	F	O	R	M	U	L	A	T	E	R	B	C	L	I	M	A	X	R	I
D	B	B	L	X	S	T	A	T	E	G	D	T	Z	S	E	V	L	E	N
E	M	D	I	A	G	R	A	M	R	A	O	U	H	O	V	T	W	D	F
N	B	E	X	W	Z	T	K	X	E	N	C	H	T	Y	E	O	V	I	E
T	C	R	E	T	E	L	L	L	L	I	H	W	F	I	N	P	P	C	R
I	M	C	F	I	M	A	F	B	I	Z	Z	U	N	E	T	W	J	T	L
F	M	O	D	I	F	I	E	R	A	E	F	C	I	A	O	R	D	E	R
Y	S	O	U	R	C	E	A	B	B	L	G	U	H	P	J	C	M	K	J
C	O	N	C	L	U	D	E	S	L	L	G	W	R	I	T	E	L	S	U
Q	Q	G	K	P	L	O	T	S	E	A	I	Z	L	J	Z	S	A	C	U
T	O	N	E	C	O	M	P	R	E	H	E	N	S	I	O	N	X	H	P

1. The moment in the story where the conflict reaches its highest point.
2. To explain an idea or make a conclusion by looking closely at evidence in text.
3. Anything that happens, especially something important or unusual.
4. Able to trust.
5. Put in order; arrange.
6. Repeat; say again.
7. To produce words.
8. To determine and mark points on a graph.
9. Sort; organize.
10. To recognize or establish as being a person or thing.
11. The meaning a reader gets from written text.
12. A writer's attitude toward his or her topic which is revealed through specific words used in the text and through figurative language.
13. To come up with.
14. A book, person, or document used to provide information or data.
15. A simplified drawing.
16. To think about carefully and form an opinion.
17. Clearly express something in a speech or writing.
18. A word, phrase or clause used to describe or qualify another word, phrase or clause.
19. Stated clearly and in detail.
20. To think of what will happen in the future or later.

A. Comprehension	B. Organize	C. Plot	D. Explicit	E. Infer
F. Tone	G. Write	H. Order	I. Identify	J. Retell
K. Diagram	L. Climax	M. Event	N. Reliable	O. Modifier
P. Predict	Q. State	R. Source	S. Concludes	T. Formulate

8. *Find the hidden words. The words have been placed horizontally, vertically, or diagonally. When you locate a word, draw a circle around it.*

O	A	W	L	B	X	Q	R	C	R	C	E	F	F	E	C	T	I	V	E
O	O	L	C	Y	L	R	E	H	E	C	V	Q	O	L	B	P	S	H	R
U	T	I	L	I	Z	E	T	A	V	O	I	A	C	D	H	V	U	T	E
I	I	M	P	A	C	T	E	R	I	L	D	X	O	Q	Q	I	S	R	S
C	J	Q	L	D	R	X	L	A	S	L	E	S	M	Y	F	S	P	A	O
P	I	U	P	L	T	N	L	C	E	E	N	J	P	K	N	U	E	C	L
I	L	L	U	S	T	R	A	T	E	C	C	B	A	J	N	A	N	E	U
P	R	E	D	I	C	T	J	E	V	T	E	S	R	H	N	L	S	W	T
N	A	R	R	A	T	O	R	R	P	C	D	H	E	Z	A	I	E	F	I
Y	Z	Z	G	O	K	E	Y	D	E	T	A	I	L	Z	R	Z	J	V	O
T	D	E	M	O	N	S	T	R	A	T	E	U	S	P	J	E	T	Z	N
D	E	F	E	N	D	M	C	P	S	R	E	L	I	A	B	L	E	W	G

1. Proof; lines and words from text used to prove or disprove an idea.
2. To make clear by using examples.
3. Imagine; think about.
4. To find similarities.
5. Support; uphold.
6. A person in a novel, play, or movie or any person, animal or figure represented in a literary work.
7. Outline; map out.
8. Helps to support the central idea in an important way. Authors elaborate using examples or anecdotes.
9. The ending, answer, or conclusion to a problem or story.
10. Able to trust.
11. Guess; tell what will happen next.
12. Change; alter.
13. A person who tells something; storyteller.
14. Repeat; say again.
15. Use something to help find a solution.
16. Show; make plain.
17. To cause changes.
18. To gather together.
19. Able to do its job to the best ability.
20. Not sure what is going to happen, waiting.

A. Character
G. Utilize
M. Compare
S. Predict

B. Effective
H. Evidence
N. Revise
T. Demonstrate

C. Resolution
I. Visualize
O. Defend

D. Trace
J. Illustrate
P. Impact

E. Collect
K. Reliable
Q. Suspense

F. Key detail
L. Narrator
R. Retell

Find the hidden words. The words have been placed horizontally, vertically, or diagonally. When you locate a word, draw a circle around it.

Q	K	R	E	L	I	A	B	L	E	J	J	R	E	V	I	S	E	V	J
C	T	O	P	I	C	M	B	V	O	R	G	A	N	I	Z	E	P	G	V
O	K	E	D	Z	C	R	E	V	E	A	L	R	S	U	M	M	A	R	Y
E	N	S	C	O	M	P	A	R	E	C	X	P	Y	N	V	D	Q	F	J
E	H	S	I	R	J	O	X	Q	U	A	N	T	I	T	A	T	I	V	E
V	E	A	I	D	I	C	O	M	P	R	E	H	E	N	S	I	O	N	C
A	C	Y	N	G	J	C	D	R	Z	C	I	M	O	D	I	F	I	E	R
L	L	O	F	F	P	L	E	I	C	L	A	S	S	I	F	Y	C	N	E
U	A	B	E	S	T	I	C	N	S	U	S	P	E	N	S	E	N	U	A
A	I	L	R	H	N	M	O	Z	V	W	L	I	X	D	E	V	G	V	T
T	M	Y	J	X	E	A	D	K	X	M	P	Z	Q	N	H	C	W	G	E
E	Q	Y	V	B	C	X	E	S	I	M	I	L	E	S	W	V	G	N	V

1. Explain how things are the same.
2. The moment in the story where the conflict reaches its highest point.
3. To show or make known.
4. Able to trust.
5. To explain an idea or make a conclusion by looking closely at evidence in text.
6. Not sure what is going to happen, waiting.
7. A word, phrase or clause used to describe or qualify another word, phrase or clause.
8. Put in order; arrange.
9. A short literary composition on a theme or subject - usually analytic or interpretive in nature.
10. Make out; break apart.
11. The subject of discussion or the subject of the article.
12. arrange (a group of people or things) in classes or categories according to shared qualities or characteristics.
13. To state a position or declare that something is true or factual, noun-a statement of truth or fact, typically pertaining to an idea that is disputed.
14. Judge; consider.
15. Data that uses characteristics.
16. Change; alter.
17. To make a product.
18. A short way of saying what the reading passage is about.
19. The meaning a reader gets from written text.
20. A comparison of two unlike things using the words "like" or "as".

A. Decode
F. Suspense
K. Create
P. Topic
B. Modifier
G. Comprehension
L. Essay
Q. Climax
C. Claim
H. Quantitative
M. Reliable
R. Organize
D. Summary
I. Reveal
N. Infer
S. Classify
E. Simile
J. Evaluate
O. Compare
T. Revise

Find the hidden words. The words have been placed horizontally, vertically, or diagonally. When you locate a word, draw a circle around it.

O	I	U	K	I	K	C	O	N	T	R	A	S	T	A	T	C	G	G	O
S	L	C	U	N	P	A	S	S	A	G	E	C	L	I	M	A	X	E	P
D	L	O	P	F	L	I	W	I	X	L	O	D	E	T	A	I	L	N	T
O	U	N	B	E	O	H	F	I	U	O	P	I	N	I	O	N	I	E	E
D	S	T	T	R	T	E	V	I	D	E	N	C	E	C	O	Q	N	R	Q
O	T	R	O	E	J	R	F	O	P	P	R	E	D	I	C	T	V	A	U
F	R	I	N	N	V	H	I	D	E	N	T	I	F	Y	O	W	A	L	J
S	A	B	E	C	M	P	A	S	S	A	G	E	U	W	N	X	L	I	V
Z	T	U	C	E	Z	S	D	E	S	Z	X	D	M	D	D	Y	I	Z	O
G	E	T	P	R	E	C	I	S	E	Q	S	I	M	I	L	E	D	E	Q
T	H	E	R	J	X	G	N	K	R	E	C	O	G	N	I	Z	E	W	P
I	F	U	N	C	T	I	O	N	K	H	O	Q	V	R	M	J	Y	B	J

1. Part; section.
2. To identify from knowledge of appearance or characteristics.
3. The events that make up the story or the main part of the story. The events relate to each other in a pattern or sequence.
4. to make a statement based upon details from the reading passage that might be true in other situations.
5. A single piece of information or fact about something.
6. To help happen or help cause.
7. Name; label.
8. The moment in the story where the conflict reaches its highest point.
9. Not true.
10. What one thinks about something or somebody.
11. A comparison of two unlike things using the words "like" or "as".
12. Proof; information in the text that proves a point.
13. Explain how things are different.
14. Exact or specific.
15. Guess; tell what will happen next.
16. Job, what it does.
17. To come up with a conclusion without valid evidence to support it.
18. To make clear by using examples.
19. A writer's attitude toward his or her topic which is revealed through specific words used in the text and through figurative language.
20. A usually short piece of written work that focuses on a topic.

A. Illustrate	B. Contribute	C. Opinion	D. Detail	E. Plot	F. Passage	G. Generalize
H. Inference	I. Identify	J. Recognize	K. Predict	L. Simile	M. Tone	N. Evidence
O. Invalid	P. Contrast	Q. Passage	R. Climax	S. Precise	T. Function	

1. *Find the hidden words. The words have been placed horizontally, vertically, or diagonally. When you locate a word, draw a circle around it.*

R	S	F	O	R	M	U	L	A	T	E	R	E	C	O	G	N	I	Z	E
C	E	D	E	S	C	R	I	B	E	V	V	N	I	N	V	A	L	I	D
K	X	O	H	Y	P	E	R	B	O	L	E	R	T	X	H	E	R	C	X
X	C	O	M	P	L	E	T	E	A	O	M	Z	O	N	H	O	V	X	F
C	O	M	P	A	R	E	E	T	S	V	C	W	N	I	L	A	K	H	U
O	D	E	S	C	R	I	B	E	S	P	R	N	E	R	Y	Y	E	H	N
L	R	E	L	I	A	B	L	E	E	B	C	L	I	M	A	X	M	X	C
T	P	V	X	F	I	E	D	L	S	I	N	T	E	R	P	R	E	T	T
O	L	J	Y	R	U	O	U	R	S	I	N	F	E	R	E	N	C	E	I
I	O	L	H	T	J	O	H	G	A	V	B	P	C	G	J	V	R	W	O
C	T	H	C	L	A	S	S	I	F	Y	Z	J	U	S	T	I	F	Y	N
C	O	N	T	R	A	S	T	S	U	P	P	O	R	T	D	D	W	H	V

1. A writer's attitude toward his or her topic which is revealed through specific words used in the text and through figurative language.
2. Judge; consider.
3. The moment in the story where the conflict reaches its highest point.
4. Give the facts; back up with details.
5. Tell how things are different; draw a distinction.
6. Finish; end.
7. Give good reason; defend.
8. To determine the meaning of.
9. Able to trust.
10. To come up with.
11. To identify from knowledge of appearance or characteristics.
12. Not true.
13. arrange (a group of people or things) in classes or categories according to shared qualities or characteristics.
14. Job, what it does.
15. The events that make up the story or the main part of the story. The events relate to each other in a pattern or sequence.
16. Tell how alike; judge against.
17. To come up with a conclusion without valid evidence to support it.
18. To tell or write about something in detail.
19. Exaggeration, not meant to be literal.
20. Tell about; explain.

A. Contrast	B. Assess	C. Climax	D. Plot
E. Interpret	F. Tone	G. Recognize	
H. Invalid	I. Inference	J. Justify	K. Formulate
L. Reliable	M. Hyperbole	N. Describe	
O. Complete	P. Classify	Q. Compare	R. Support
S. Function	T. Describe		

2. *Find the hidden words. The words have been placed horizontally, vertically, or diagonally. When you locate a word, draw a circle around it.*

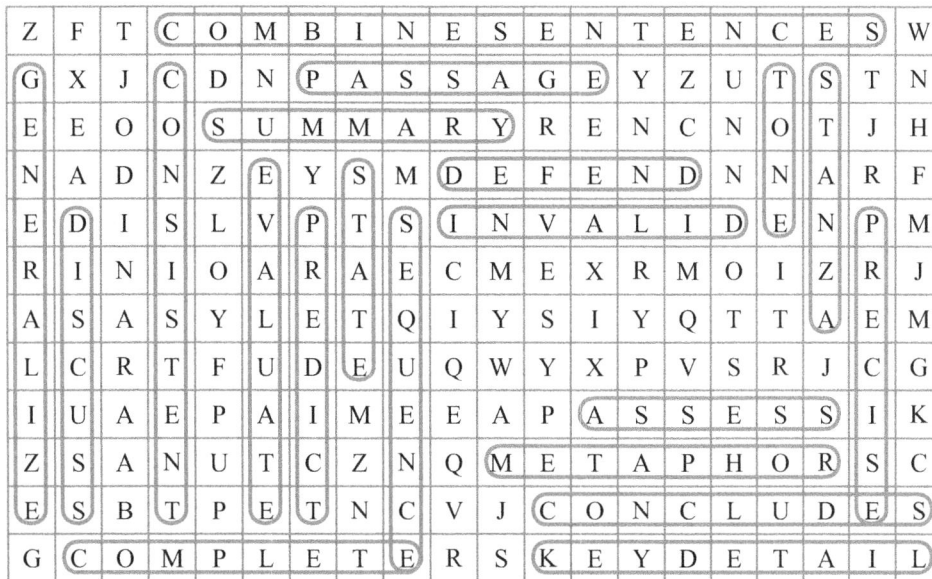

Z	F	T	C	O	M	B	I	N	E	S	E	N	T	E	N	C	E	S	W
G	X	J	C	D	N	P	A	S	S	A	G	E	Y	Z	U	T	S	T	N
E	E	O	O	S	U	M	M	A	R	Y	R	E	N	C	N	O	T	J	H
N	A	D	N	Z	E	Y	S	M	D	E	F	E	N	D	N	N	A	R	F
E	D	I	S	L	V	P	T	S	I	N	V	A	L	I	D	E	N	P	M
R	I	N	I	O	A	R	A	E	C	M	E	X	R	M	O	I	Z	R	J
A	S	A	S	Y	L	E	T	Q	I	Y	S	I	Y	Q	T	T	A	E	M
L	C	R	T	F	U	D	E	U	Q	W	Y	X	P	V	S	R	J	C	G
I	U	A	E	P	A	I	M	E	E	A	P	A	S	S	E	S	S	I	K
Z	S	A	N	U	T	C	Z	N	Q	M	E	T	A	P	H	O	R	S	C
E	S	B	T	P	E	T	N	C	V	J	C	O	N	C	L	U	D	E	S
G	C	O	M	P	L	E	T	E	R	S	K	E	Y	D	E	T	A	I	L

1. Guess; tell what will happen next.
2. A writer's attitude toward his or her topic which is revealed through specific words used in the text and through figurative language.
3. A short way of saying what the reading passage is about.
4. A comparison of two unlike things by describing one is the other.
5. Say; affirm.
6. to make a statement based upon details from the reading passage that might be true in other situations.
7. Support; uphold.
8. A usually short piece of written work that focuses on a topic.
9. To judge or determine the quality or amount of something.
10. A group of lines forming the basic unit in a poem; a verse.
11. Helps to support the central idea in an important way. Authors elaborate using examples or anecdotes.
12. Finish; end.
13. To consider an idea.
14. To merge two or more sentences into one sentence.
15. To do something the same constantly.
16. Judge; consider.
17. Order in which events, movements, or things follow each other.
18. Exact or specific.
19. To think about carefully and form an opinion.
20. Not true.

A. Stanza	B. Sequence	C. Metaphor	D. Evaluate	E. Complete
F. Discuss	G. Tone	H. Invalid	I. Combine sentences	J. Concludes
K. Defend	L. State	M. Assess	N. Predict	O. Consistent
P. Passage	Q. Generalize	R. Summary	S. Key detail	T. Precise

3. *Find the hidden words. The words have been placed horizontally, vertically, or diagonally. When you locate a word, draw a circle around it.*

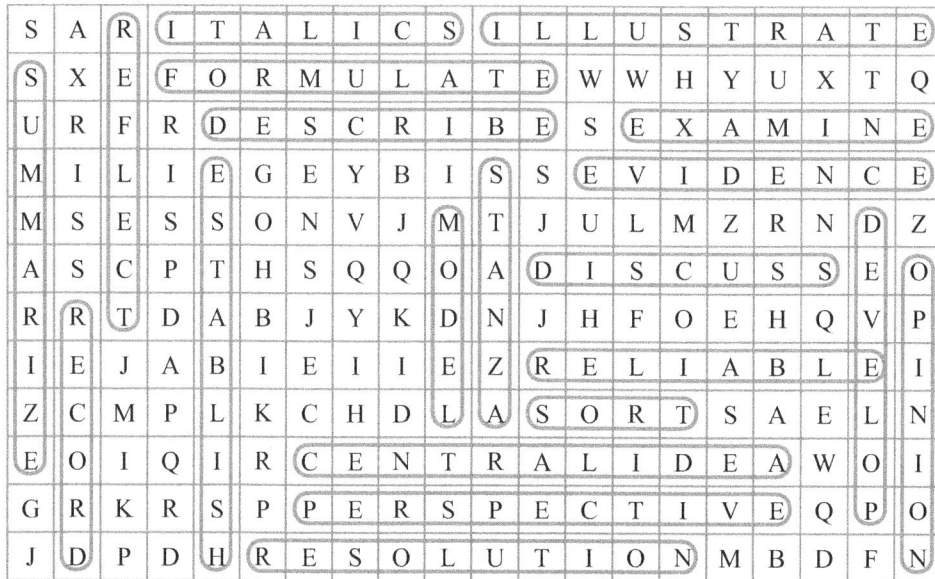

S	A	R	I	T	A	L	I	C	S	I	L	L	U	S	T	R	A	T	E
S	X	E	F	O	R	M	U	L	A	T	E	W	W	H	Y	U	X	T	Q
U	R	F	R	D	E	S	C	R	I	B	E	S	E	X	A	M	I	N	E
M	I	I	E	G	E	Y	B	I	S	S	E	V	I	D	E	N	C	E
M	S	E	S	S	O	N	V	J	M	T	J	U	L	M	Z	R	N	D	Z
A	S	C	P	T	H	S	Q	Q	O	A	D	I	S	C	U	S	S	E	O
R	R	T	D	A	B	J	Y	K	D	N	J	H	F	O	E	H	Q	V	P
I	E	J	A	B	I	E	I	I	E	Z	R	E	L	I	A	B	L	E	I
Z	C	M	P	L	K	C	H	D	L	A	S	O	R	T	S	A	E	L	N
E	O	I	Q	I	R	C	E	N	T	R	A	L	I	D	E	A	W	O	I
G	R	K	R	S	P	P	E	R	S	P	E	C	T	I	V	E	Q	P	O
J	D	P	D	H	R	E	S	O	L	U	T	I	O	N	M	B	D	F	N

1. Group; classify.
2. A group of lines forming the basic unit in a poem; a verse.
3. To show to be true, to prove.
4. Talk about; argue.
5. To tell or write about something in detail.
6. Proof; lines and words from text used to prove or disprove an idea.
7. To put down in writing so that it is saved.
8. The ending, answer, or conclusion to a problem or story.
9. What the passage or text is mainly about.
10. To draw or make pictures to explain.
11. Put together; create.
12. To paraphrase or to explain in your own words an important idea or section of text.
13. Think about; wonder about.
14. Look at; inspect.
15. An opinion or the way someone looks at something.
16. A style of print where the letters slope to the right; may be used to emphasize or to indicate the title of published work.
17. What one thinks about something or somebody.
18. To work out, grow, or expand.
19. To represent something that will serve as an example.
20. Able to trust.

A. Reflect
B. Opinion
C. Establish
D. Record
E. Illustrate
F. Describe
G. Central idea
H. Sort
I. Resolution
J. Italics
K. Summarize
L. Perspective
M. Model
N. Evidence
O. Reliable
P. Stanza
Q. Develop
R. Discuss
S. Formulate
T. Examine

4. *Find the hidden words. The words have been placed horizontally, vertically, or diagonally. When you locate a word, draw a circle around it.*

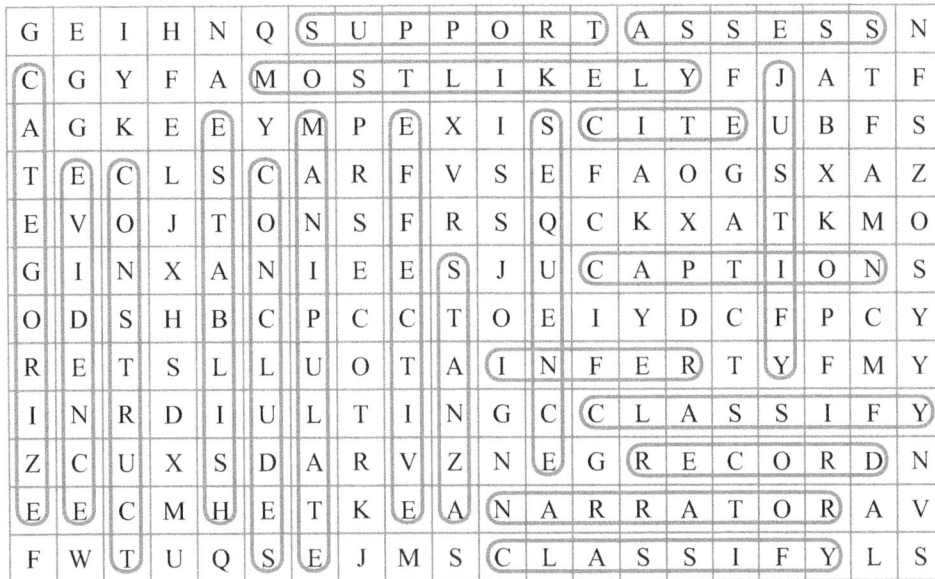

G	E	I	H	N	Q	S	U	P	P	O	R	T	A	S	S	E	S	S	N
C	G	Y	F	A	M	O	S	T	L	I	K	E	L	Y	F	J	A	T	F
A	G	K	E	E	Y	M	P	E	X	I	S	C	I	T	E	U	B	F	S
T	E	C	L	S	C	A	R	F	V	S	E	F	A	O	G	S	X	A	Z
E	V	O	J	T	O	N	S	F	R	S	Q	C	K	X	A	T	K	M	O
G	I	N	X	A	N	I	E	E	S	J	U	C	A	P	T	I	O	N	S
O	D	S	H	B	C	P	C	C	T	O	E	I	Y	D	C	F	P	C	Y
R	E	T	S	L	L	U	O	T	A	I	N	F	E	R	T	Y	F	M	Y
I	N	R	D	I	U	L	T	I	N	G	C	C	L	A	S	S	I	F	Y
Z	C	U	X	S	D	A	R	V	Z	N	E	G	R	E	C	O	R	D	N
E	E	C	M	H	E	T	K	E	A	N	A	R	R	A	T	O	R	A	V
F	W	T	U	Q	S	E	J	M	S	C	L	A	S	S	I	F	Y	L	S

1. Will probably happen; probably.
2. A group of lines forming the basic unit in a poem; a verse.
3. To prove.
4. Able to do its job to the best ability.
5. To think about carefully and form an opinion.
6. Place in a class or group.
7. An explanation for a picture or illustration.
8. To show to be true, to prove.
9. Put in order; sort.
10. arrange (a group of people or things) in classes or categories according to shared qualities or characteristics.
11. Proof; lines and words from text used to prove or disprove an idea.
12. To use a quote from the text to support an idea.
13. A person who tells something; storyteller.
14. To put down in writing so that it is saved.
15. To change something to work in a certain way.
16. Make a good guess; read between the lines.
17. Judge; consider.
18. Order in which events, movements, or things follow each other.
19. To make a product.
20. To provide proof or evidence for.

A. Support	B. Construct	C. Effective	D. Sequence	E. Infer	F. Establish	G. Concludes
H. Caption	I. Evidence	J. Record	K. Justify	L. Assess	M. Narrator	N. Most likely
O. Cite	P. Manipulate	Q. Stanza	R. Categorize	S. Classify	T. Classify	

5. *Find the hidden words. The words have been placed horizontally, vertically, or diagonally. When you locate a word, draw a circle around it.*

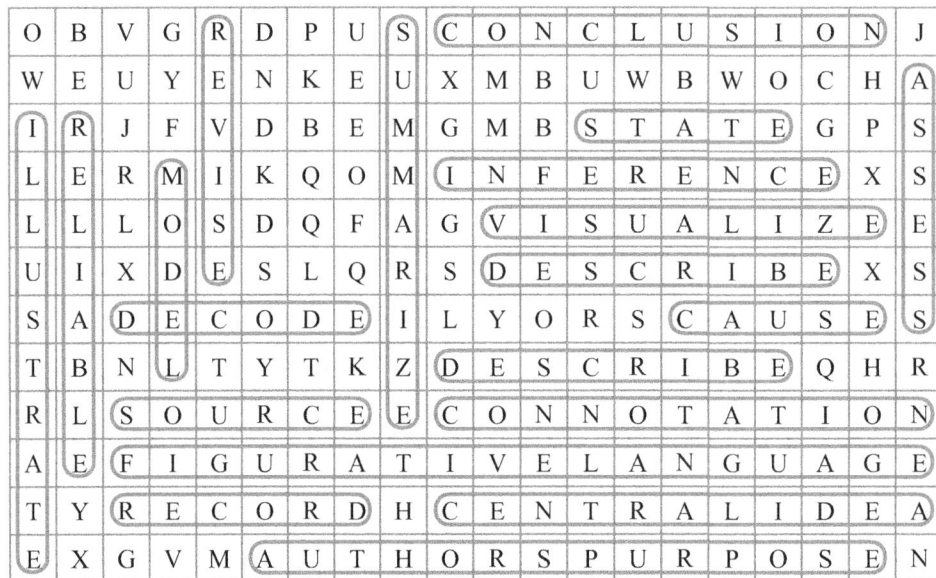

O	B	V	G	R	D	P	U	S	C	O	N	C	L	U	S	I	O	N	J
W	E	U	Y	E	N	K	E	U	X	M	B	U	W	B	W	O	C	H	A
I	R	J	F	V	D	B	E	M	G	M	B	S	T	A	T	E	G	P	S
L	E	R	M	I	K	Q	O	M	I	N	F	E	R	E	N	C	E	X	S
L	L	L	O	S	D	Q	F	A	G	V	I	S	U	A	L	I	Z	E	E
U	I	X	D	E	S	L	Q	R	S	D	E	S	C	R	I	B	E	X	S
S	A	D	E	C	O	D	E	I	L	Y	O	R	S	C	A	U	S	E	S
T	B	N	L	T	Y	T	K	Z	D	E	S	C	R	I	B	E	Q	H	R
R	L	S	O	U	R	C	E	C	O	N	N	O	T	A	T	I	O	N
A	E	F	I	G	U	R	A	T	I	V	E	L	A	N	G	U	A	G	E
T	Y	R	E	C	O	R	D	H	C	E	N	T	R	A	L	I	D	E	A
E	X	G	V	M	A	U	T	H	O	R	S	P	U	R	P	O	S	E	N

1. Change; alter.
2. To make clear by using examples.
3. Sum it up; give a short version.
4. To tell or write about something in detail.
5. Ending; wrapping up.
6. Judge; consider.
7. The reason why something happens.
8. Reason the author writes: persuade, inform, entertain (PIE).
9. Imagine; think about.
10. Make out; break apart.
11. To tell the facts, details.
12. To represent something that will serve as an example.
13. A conclusion reached based on reasoning and the use of given facts; a prediction.
14. Say; affirm.
15. Able to trust.
16. All the meanings, associations, emotions, or tones that a word suggests.
17. A book, person, or document used to provide information or data.
18. Words that may not literally mean what they say.
19. To put down in writing so that it is saved.
20. What the passage or text is mainly about.

A. Authors purpose
B. Illustrate
C. Central idea
D. Connotation
E. Source
F. Reliable
G. Describe
H. Model
I. State
J. Assess
K. Conclusion
L. Cause
M. Figurative language
N. Record
O. Inference
P. Summarize
Q. Visualize
R. Describe
S. Decode
T. Revise

6. *Find the hidden words. The words have been placed horizontally, vertically, or diagonally. When you locate a word, draw a circle around it.*

S	S	S	M	O	D	I	F	I	E	R	V	M	W	L	X	F	I	E	W
O	E	U	K	Q	T	N	I	G	R	E	T	E	L	L	U	O	M	X	O
U	Q	P	R	R	W	J	E	R	R	U	O	U	T	L	I	N	E	A	R
R	U	P	E	E	N	U	V	S	E	Q	U	E	N	C	E	W	Y	G	E
C	E	O	V	S	D	S	G	R	Y	Z	L	C	P	D	F	B	A	G	F
E	N	R	I	U	E	T	T	E	X	T	Z	O	S	D	B	D	T	E	E
U	C	T	S	L	S	I	M	L	E	W	O	N	T	E	T	D	T	R	R
Q	E	D	I	T	C	F	Y	I	K	E	T	V	A	F	O	K	I	A	E
S	Y	I	O	W	R	Y	E	A	S	I	P	E	T	I	P	A	T	T	N
H	C	Y	N	K	I	E	D	B	J	D	E	Y	E	N	I	V	U	I	C
M	J	U	K	Z	B	U	C	L	R	X	R	N	E	C	C	D	O	E
F	P	T	R	U	E	J	X	E	G	T	N	T	F	C	Y	D	E	N	Y

1. To prove.
2. Put in order; put in a series.
3. The subject of discussion or the subject of the article.
4. Give an answer; consequence.
5. Give the facts; back up with details.
6. Describe; characterize.
7. A book, person, or document used to provide information or data.
8. To connect back to another text.
9. The reading passage.
10. To make things or ideas known to others; to share or to get ideas across to others.
11. Able to trust.
12. Give a rough idea; plan.
13. A word, phrase or clause used to describe or qualify another word, phrase or clause.
14. Order in which events, movements, or things follow each other.
15. The fact of making something seem larger, more important, better, or worse than it really is; overstate the truth.
16. Tell about; explain.
17. Repeat; say again.
18. A corrected or new version of something written.
19. Clearly express something in a speech or writing.
20. The way someone feels about something.

A. Attitude	B. Justify	C. Exaggeration	D. Support
G. Sequence	H. Define	I. Reliable	J. Outline
M. Retell	N. Result	O. Text	P. State
S. Topic	T. Reference		

E. Revision   F. Convey
K. Source   L. Modifier
Q. Describe   R. Sequence

7. *Find the hidden words. The words have been placed horizontally, vertically, or diagonally. When you locate a word, draw a circle around it.*

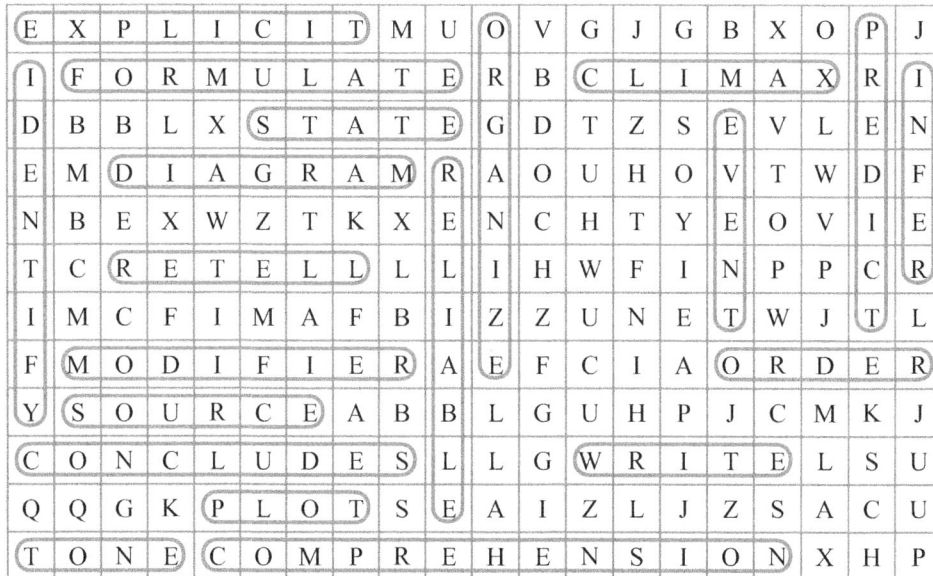

E	X	P	L	I	C	I	T	M	U	O	V	G	J	G	B	X	O	P	J
I	F	O	R	M	U	L	A	T	E	R	B	C	L	I	M	A	X	R	I
D	B	B	L	X	S	T	A	T	E	G	D	T	Z	S	E	V	L	E	N
E	M	D	I	A	G	R	A	M	R	A	O	U	H	O	V	T	W	D	F
N	B	E	X	W	Z	T	K	X	E	N	C	H	T	Y	E	O	V	I	E
T	C	R	E	T	E	L	L	L	L	I	H	W	F	I	N	P	P	C	R
I	M	C	F	I	M	A	F	B	I	Z	Z	U	N	E	T	W	J	T	L
F	M	O	D	I	F	I	E	R	A	E	F	C	I	A	O	R	D	E	R
Y	S	O	U	R	C	E	A	B	B	L	G	U	H	P	J	C	M	K	J
C	O	N	C	L	U	D	E	S	L	L	G	W	R	I	T	E	L	S	U
Q	Q	G	K	P	L	O	T	S	E	A	I	Z	L	J	Z	S	A	C	U
T	O	N	E	C	O	M	P	R	E	H	E	N	S	I	O	N	X	H	P

1. The moment in the story where the conflict reaches its highest point.
2. To explain an idea or make a conclusion by looking closely at evidence in text.
3. Anything that happens, especially something important or unusual.
4. Able to trust.
5. Put in order; arrange.
6. Repeat; say again.
7. To produce words.
8. To determine and mark points on a graph.
9. Sort; organize.
10. To recognize or establish as being a person or thing.
11. The meaning a reader gets from written text.
12. A writer's attitude toward his or her topic which is revealed through specific words used in the text and through figurative language.
13. To come up with.
14. A book, person, or document used to provide information or data.
15. A simplified drawing.
16. To think about carefully and form an opinion.
17. Clearly express something in a speech or writing.
18. A word, phrase or clause used to describe or qualify another word, phrase or clause.
19. Stated clearly and in detail.
20. To think of what will happen in the future or later.

A. Comprehension	B. Organize	C. Plot	D. Explicit	E. Infer
F. Tone	G. Write	H. Order	I. Identify	J. Retell
K. Diagram	L. Climax	M. Event	N. Reliable	O. Modifier
P. Predict	Q. State	R. Source	S. Concludes	T. Formulate

8. *Find the hidden words. The words have been placed horizontally, vertically, or diagonally. When you locate a word, draw a circle around it.*

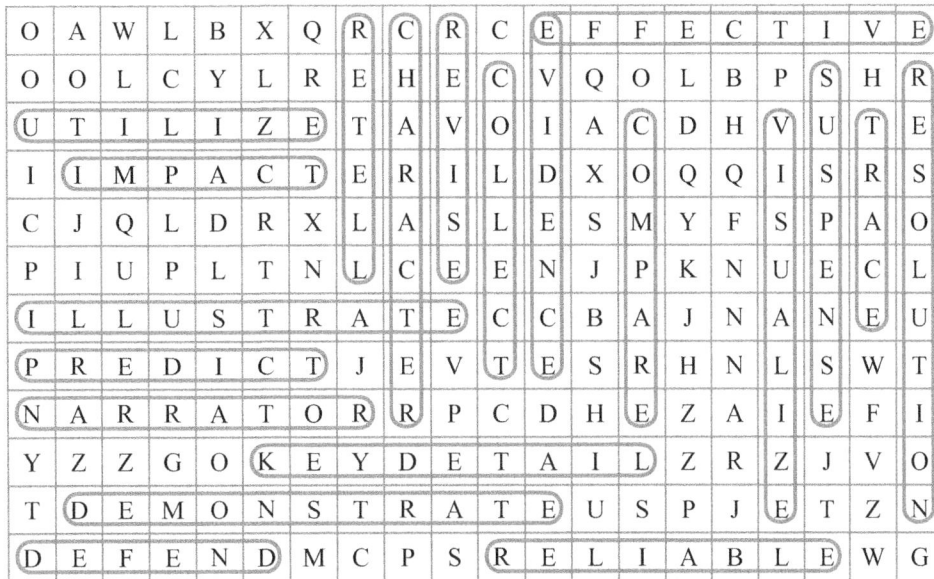

O	A	W	L	B	X	Q	R	C	R	C	E	F	F	E	C	T	I	V	E
O	O	L	C	Y	L	R	E	H	E	C	V	Q	O	L	B	P	S	H	R
U	T	I	L	I	Z	E	T	A	V	O	I	A	C	D	H	V	U	T	E
I	I	M	P	A	C	T	E	R	I	L	D	X	O	Q	Q	I	S	R	S
C	J	Q	L	D	R	X	L	A	S	L	E	S	M	Y	F	S	P	A	O
P	I	U	P	L	T	N	L	C	E	E	N	J	P	K	N	U	E	C	L
I	L	L	U	S	T	R	A	T	E	C	C	B	A	J	N	A	N	E	U
P	R	E	D	I	C	T	J	E	V	T	E	S	R	H	N	L	S	W	T
N	A	R	R	A	T	O	R	R	P	C	D	H	E	Z	A	I	E	F	I
Y	Z	Z	G	O	K	E	Y	D	E	T	A	I	L	Z	R	Z	J	V	O
T	D	E	M	O	N	S	T	R	A	T	E	U	S	P	J	E	T	Z	N
D	E	F	E	N	D	M	C	P	S	R	E	L	I	A	B	L	E	W	G

1. Proof; lines and words from text used to prove or disprove an idea.
2. To make clear by using examples.
3. Imagine; think about.
4. To find similarities.
5. Support; uphold.
6. A person in a novel, play, or movie or any person, animal or figure represented in a literary work.
7. Outline; map out.
8. Helps to support the central idea in an important way. Authors elaborate using examples or anecdotes.
9. The ending, answer, or conclusion to a problem or story.
10. Able to trust.
11. Guess; tell what will happen next.
12. Change; alter.
13. A person who tells something; storyteller.
14. Repeat; say again.
15. Use something to help find a solution.
16. Show; make plain.
17. To cause changes.
18. To gather together.
19. Able to do its job to the best ability.
20. Not sure what is going to happen, waiting.

A. Character
B. Effective
C. Resolution
D. Trace
E. Collect
F. Key detail
G. Utilize
H. Evidence
I. Visualize
J. Illustrate
K. Reliable
L. Narrator
M. Compare
N. Revise
O. Defend
P. Impact
Q. Suspense
R. Retell
S. Predict
T. Demonstrate

9. *Find the hidden words. The words have been placed horizontally, vertically, or diagonally. When you locate a word, draw a circle around it.*

Q	K	R	E	L	I	A	B	L	E	J	J	R	E	V	I	S	E	V	J
C	T	O	P	I	C	M	B	V	O	R	G	A	N	I	Z	E	P	G	V
O	K	E	D	Z	C	R	E	V	E	A	L	R	S	U	M	M	A	R	Y
E	N	S	C	O	M	P	A	R	E	C	X	P	Y	N	V	D	Q	F	J
E	H	S	I	R	J	O	X	Q	U	A	N	T	I	T	A	T	I	V	E
V	E	A	I	D	I	C	O	M	P	R	E	H	E	N	S	I	O	N	C
A	C	Y	N	G	J	C	D	R	Z	C	I	M	O	D	I	F	I	E	R
L	L	O	F	F	P	L	E	I	C	L	A	S	S	I	F	Y	C	N	E
U	A	B	E	S	T	I	C	N	S	U	S	P	E	N	S	E	N	U	A
A	I	L	R	H	N	M	O	Z	V	W	L	I	X	D	E	V	G	V	T
T	M	Y	J	X	E	A	D	K	X	M	P	Z	Q	N	H	C	W	G	E
E	Q	Y	V	B	C	X	E	S	I	M	I	L	E	S	W	V	G	N	V

1. Explain how things are the same.
2. The moment in the story where the conflict reaches its highest point.
3. To show or make known.
4. Able to trust.
5. To explain an idea or make a conclusion by looking closely at evidence in text.
6. Not sure what is going to happen, waiting.
7. A word, phrase or clause used to describe or qualify another word, phrase or clause.
8. Put in order; arrange.
9. A short literary composition on a theme or subject - usually analytic or interpretive in nature.
10. Make out; break apart.
11. The subject of discussion or the subject of the article.
12. arrange (a group of people or things) in classes or categories according to shared qualities or characteristics.
13. To state a position or declare that something is true or factual, noun-a statement of truth or fact, typically pertaining to an idea that is disputed.
14. Judge; consider.
15. Data that uses characteristics.
16. Change; alter.
17. To make a product.
18. A short way of saying what the reading passage is about.
19. The meaning a reader gets from written text.
20. A comparison of two unlike things using the words "like" or "as".

A. Decode	B. Modifier	C. Claim	D. Summary	E. Simile
F. Suspense	G. Comprehension	H. Quantitative	I. Reveal	J. Evaluate
K. Create	L. Essay	M. Reliable	N. Infer	O. Compare
P. Topic	Q. Climax	R. Organize	S. Classify	T. Revise

10. *Find the hidden words. The words have been placed horizontally, vertically, or diagonally. When you locate a word, draw a circle around it.*

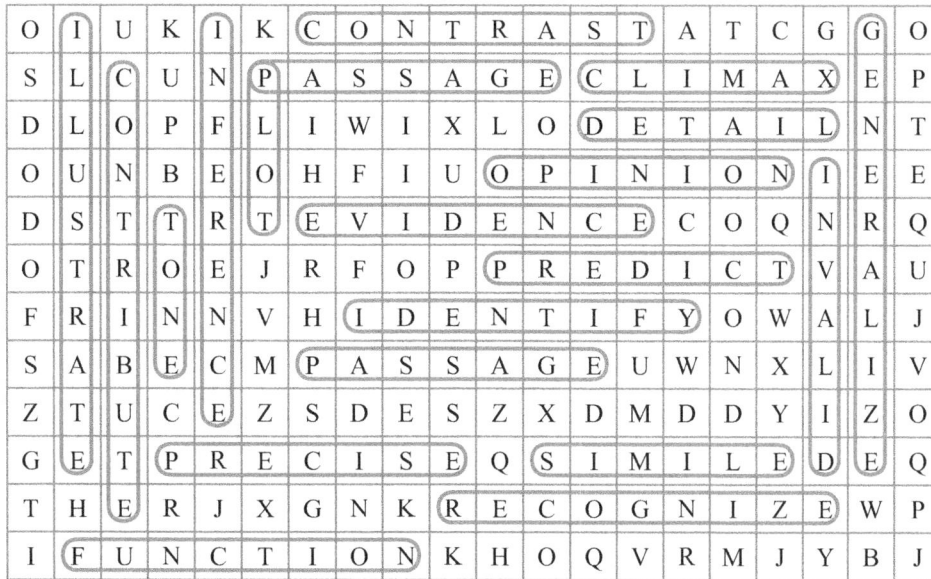

O	I	U	K	I	K	C	O	N	T	R	A	S	T	A	T	C	G	G	O
S	L	C	U	N	P	A	S	S	A	G	E	C	L	I	M	A	X	E	P
D	L	O	P	F	L	I	W	I	X	L	O	D	E	T	A	I	L	N	T
O	U	N	B	E	O	H	F	I	U	O	P	I	N	I	O	N	I	E	E
D	S	T	T	R	T	E	V	I	D	E	N	C	E	C	O	Q	N	R	Q
O	T	R	O	E	J	R	F	O	P	P	R	E	D	I	C	T	V	A	U
F	R	I	N	N	V	H	I	D	E	N	T	I	F	Y	O	W	A	L	J
S	A	B	E	C	M	P	A	S	S	A	G	E	U	W	N	X	L	I	V
Z	T	U	C	E	Z	S	D	E	S	Z	X	D	M	D	D	Y	I	Z	O
G	E	T	P	R	E	C	I	S	E	Q	S	I	M	I	L	E	D	E	Q
T	H	E	R	J	X	G	N	K	R	E	C	O	G	N	I	Z	E	W	P
I	F	U	N	C	T	I	O	N	K	H	O	Q	V	R	M	J	Y	B	J

1. Part; section.
2. To identify from knowledge of appearance or characteristics.
3. The events that make up the story or the main part of the story. The events relate to each other in a pattern or sequence.
4. to make a statement based upon details from the reading passage that might be true in other situations.
5. A single piece of information or fact about something.
6. To help happen or help cause.
7. Name; label.
8. The moment in the story where the conflict reaches its highest point.
9. Not true.
10. What one thinks about something or somebody.
11. A comparison of two unlike things using the words "like" or "as".
12. Proof; information in the text that proves a point.
13. Explain how things are different.
14. Exact or specific.
15. Guess; tell what will happen next.
16. Job, what it does.
17. To come up with a conclusion without valid evidence to support it.
18. To make clear by using examples.
19. A writer's attitude toward his or her topic which is revealed through specific words used in the text and through figurative language.
20. A usually short piece of written work that focuses on a topic.

A. Illustrate	B. Contribute	C. Opinion	D. Detail	E. Plot	F. Passage	G. Generalize
H. Inference	I. Identify	J. Recognize	K. Predict	L. Simile	M. Tone	N. Evidence
O. Invalid	P. Contrast	Q. Passage	R. Climax	S. Precise	T. Function	

Glossary

Analysis of text: Read and examine text in detail looking for important ideas.

Analyze: Break apart; study the pieces.

Analyze: To look at text carefully by paying attention to its parts, its words, its figurative language, and its tone.

Apply: To use.

Assess: Judge; consider.

Associate: To relate to concepts.

Attitude: The way someone feels about something.

Authors purpose: Reason the author writes- persuade, inform, entertain (PIE).

Best: Above all others, most desirable.

Calculate: Work out; compute.

Caption: An explanation for a picture or illustration.

Categorize: Place in a class or group.

Categorize: To put in a group based on certain characteristics.

Cause: The reason why something happens.

Central idea: The main point of the story or the text; the unifying element of a story or text, sometimes called main idea or theme.

Central idea: What the passage or text is mainly about.

Character: A person in a novel, play, or movie or any person, animal or figure represented in a literary work.

Cite: To use a quote from the text to support an idea.

Claim: To state a position or declare that something is true or factual, noun-a statement of truth or fact, typically pertaining to an idea that is disputed.

Classify: arrange (a group of people or things) in classes or categories according to shared qualities or characteristics.

Classify: Put in order; sort.

Climax: The moment in the story where the conflict reaches its highest point.

Collect: To gather together.

Combine sentences: To merge two or more sentences into one sentence.

Compare: Explain how things are the same.

Compare: Tell how alike; judge against.

Compare: To find similarities.

Complete: Finish; end.

Comprehension: The meaning a reader gets from written text.

Conclude: to decide based upon information stated in the reading passages.

Concludes: To think about carefully and form an opinion.

Concluding sentence: A sentence that pulls together or summarizes the main idea and provides a definite ending point for a paragraph or written piece.

Conclusion: Ending; wrapping up.

Connotation: All the meanings, associations, emotions, or tones that a word suggests.

Consistent: To do something the same constantly.

Construct: To make a product.

Contrast: Explain how things are different.

Contrast: Tell how things are different; draw a distinction.

Contrast: To find differences.

Contribute: To help happen or help cause.

Convey: To make things or ideas known to others; to share or to get ideas across to others.

Convince: To persuade or get someone to think a certain way.

Create: To make a product.

Decode: Make out; break apart.

Defend: Support; uphold.

Define: Describe; characterize.

Demonstrate: Show; make plain.

Denotation: The basic definition or dictionary meaning of a word.

Describe: Tell about; explain.

Describe: To tell or write about something in detail.

Describe: To tell the facts, details.

Detail: A single piece of information or fact about something.

Details: Provide exact items; be specific.

Determine: To decide.

Develop: To work out, grow, or expand.

Diagram: A simplified drawing.

Diagram: Label the parts of the drawing; make a drawing, chart, or plan.

Discuss: Talk about; argue.

Discuss: To consider an idea.

Distinguish: To tell as different.

Draft: Plain; rough copy.

Effect: What happens because of something.

Effective: Able to do its job to the best ability.

Enclosed: To include with something else (e.g. the money is enclosed with the letter in the envelope); to close or hold in.

Essay: A short literary composition on a theme or subject - usually analytic or interpretive in nature.

Establish: To show to be true, to prove.

Evaluate: Judge; consider.

Evaluate: To judge or determine the quality or amount of something.

Event: Anything that happens, especially something important or unusual.

Evidence: Proof; information in the text that proves a point.

Evidence: Proof; lines and words from text used to prove or disprove an idea.

Exaggeration: The fact of making something seem larger, more important, better, or worse than it really is; overstate the truth.

Examine: Look at; inspect.

Example: Give an instance; case.

Excerpt: A part of a reading passage.

Explain: Make clear; put in your own words.

Explain: To give details to make something clear.

Explain: To make known in detail.

Explicit: Stated clearly and in detail.

Figurative language: Words or expression different from literal language, changed or altered to make a linguistic point.

Figurative language: Words that may not literally mean what they say.

Formulate: Put together; create.

Formulate: To come up with.

Function: Job, what it does.

Generalize: to make a statement based upon details from the reading passage that might be true in other situations.

Hyperbole: Exaggeration, not meant to be literal.

Identify: Name; label.

Identify: To recognize or establish as being a person or thing.

Illustrate: To draw or make pictures to explain.

Illustrate: To make clear by using examples.

Image: A form of figurative language and descriptive language that creates a picture in your mind.

Impact: To cause changes.

Imply: to hint at something without saying it.

Infer: Make a good guess; read between the lines.

Infer: To explain an idea or make a conclusion by looking closely at evidence in text.

Inference: A conclusion reached based on reasoning and the use of given facts; a prediction.

Inference: To come up with a conclusion without valid evidence to support it.

Interpret: Explain the meaning; make clear.

Interpret: To determine the meaning of.

Invalid: Not true.

Investigate: To search for an answer to a solution.

Italics: A style of print where the letters slope to the right; may be used to emphasize or to indicate the title of published work.

Justify: Give good reason; defend.

Justify: To prove.

Key detail: Helps to support the central idea in an important way. Authors elaborate using examples or anecdotes.

Label: Name; identify.

List: Record; name.

Manipulate: To change something to work in a certain way.

Metaphor: A comparison of two unlike things by describing one is the other.

Model: To represent something that will serve as an example.

Modifier: A word, phrase or clause used to describe or qualify another word, phrase or clause.

Mood: A temporary state of mind or feeling.

Most likely: Will probably happen; probably.

Narrative: A story.

Narrator: A person who tells something; storyteller.

Observe: Watch; notice.

Opinion: What one thinks about something or somebody.

Order: Sort; organize.

Organize: Put in order; arrange.

Outline: Give a rough idea; plan.

Paragraph: A section of writing consisting of one or more sentences grouped together and discussing one main subject.

Paraphrase: A restatement of the meaning of a text or passage using other words.

Passage: A usually short piece of written work that focuses on a topic.

Passage: Part; section.

Perspective: An opinion or the way someone looks at something.

Phrase: A group of words within a text.

Plot: The events that make up the story or the main part of the story. The events relate to each other in a pattern or sequence.

Plot: To determine and mark points on a graph.

Precise: Exact or specific.

Predict: Guess; tell what will happen next.

Predict: To think of what will happen in the future or later.

Purpose: The reason someone does something.

Qualitative: Data that is based on numbers.

Quantitative: Data that uses characteristics.

Quotation mark: A punctuation mark ", " or ',' used at the beginning and ending of text that has been stated from a source.

Recognize: To identify from knowledge of appearance or characteristics.

Record: To put down in writing so that it is saved.

Reference: To connect back to another text.

Reflect: Think about; wonder about.

Reliable: Able to trust.

Reproduce: Copy; repeat.

Resolution: The ending, answer, or conclusion to a problem or story.

Response: An answer or reply.

Restate: Repeat; say again.

Result: Give an answer; consequence.

Retell: Repeat; say again.

Reveal: To show or make known.

Review: Look at; study.

Revise: Change; alter.

Revision: A corrected or new version of something written.

Select: To choose.

Sequence: Order in which events, movements, or things follow each other.

Sequence: Put in order; put in a series.

Setting: The period and-or location in which a story takes place.

Significance: A part of the story that is important.

Simile: A comparison of two unlike things using the words "like" or "as".

Sort: Group; classify.

Source: A book, person, or document used to provide information or data.

Stanza: A group of lines forming the basic unit in a poem; a verse.

Stanza: A group of lines in a poem (similar to a paragraph).

State: Clearly express something in a speech or writing.

State: Say; affirm.

Summarize: Sum it up; give a short version.

Summarize: To paraphrase or to explain in your own words an important idea or section of text.

Summary: A short way of saying what the reading passage is about.

Summary: Using few words to give the most important information about something or a complete but brief account of things previously stated.

Support: Give the facts; back up with details.

Support: To provide proof or evidence for.

Support: Use details from the text to explain your response.

Suspense: Not sure what is going to happen, waiting.

Text structure: The way a text is presented- introduction, headings and subheads, sentences that form paragraphs, and chapters.

Text: A book or other written work or printed work.

Text: The reading passage.

Textual evidence: Text that the author presents as an argument.

Tone: A writer's attitude toward his or her topic which is revealed through specific words used in the text and through figurative language.

Topic: The subject of discussion or the subject of the article.

Trace: Outline; map out.

Utilize: Use something to help find a solution.

Valid: True.

Viewpoint: A way of looking or thinking about something.

Visualize: Imagine; think about.

Write: To produce words.

Made in the USA
Las Vegas, NV
10 February 2022